HERBOLUTION

HERBOLUTION

New Discoveries in Detoxification Using Herbal Enzymes

Kevin Sullivan, N.D.

TATE PUBLISHING & *Enterprises*

Herbolution
Copyright © 2011 by Kevin Sullivan, N.D.. All rights reserved.

No part of this publication may be reproduced, stored in a retrieval system or transmitted in any way by any means, electronic, mechanical, photocopy, recording or otherwise without the prior permission of the author except as provided by USA copyright law.

Scripture quotations are taken from the *Holy Bible, King James Version*, Cambridge, 1769. Used by permission. All rights reserved.

The opinions expressed by the author are not necessarily those of Tate Publishing, LLC.

Published by Tate Publishing & Enterprises, LLC
127 E. Trade Center Terrace | Mustang, Oklahoma 73064 USA
1.888.361.9473 | www.tatepublishing.com

Tate Publishing is committed to excellence in the publishing industry. The company reflects the philosophy established by the founders, based on Psalm 68:11,
"The Lord gave the word and great was the company of those who published it."

Book design copyright © 2011 by Tate Publishing, LLC. All rights reserved.
Cover design by Joey Garrett
Interior design by Chelsea Womble

Published in the United States of America

ISBN: 978-1-60604-901-3
1. Health & Fitness, Homeopathy
2. Health & Fitness, Herbal Medications
11.05.04

From the Bible, *Luke 4:23* (King James Version):

> "And he said unto them, Ye will surely say unto me this proverb, Physician, heal thyself: whatsoever we have heard done in Capernaum, do also here in thy country."

The information presented in this book is based on the opinions, theories, research, and training of the author. This book is not intended as medical advice, nor is it intended to replace the advice or prescribed treatment of anyone's practitioner. The purpose of the information contained in this book is only education. The author has made every effort to present the information in this book accurately and assumes no responsibility for inaccuracies. The author is not liable for any misuse of the information provided. Consult a qualified health professional for the appropriate advice and treatment options available before starting any new health regimen.

TABLE OF CONTENTS

Acknowledgments 11
Introduction.. 13
Of Course You Have Toxins!.. 17

TOXINS

<u>ORGANIC TOXINS</u>
Of Course You Have Parasites! 23
Bacteria, Fungi and Viruses..25
Autism 29
Venoms... 31

<u>INORGANIC TOXINS</u>
Chemicals 33

Final Thoughts on Toxins..37

REMEDIES

Homeopathy 41
Herbs and Metabolic Enzymes......................................45
The Importance of Cofactors 49
Miasms 51
Endocrine Glands 53
The Successful Solution 55

Symptom List 61
Nutrition in Your Diet 63
Athletic Performance 69
Aging 73
Biblical Perspective 75
Final Thoughts on Remedies 83

NUTRIENTS

Enzymes 87
Vitamins 111
Minerals 115
Trace Elements 121
Amino Acids 127
Phenolics 133
Nutritional Recommendations 143
Nutrient Superstars 173
Final Thoughts 187
Conclusion 193

References 195

ACKNOWLEDGMENTS

I want to thank everyone involved in creating this book. First, to my dear wife Laura, who supported and encouraged me in this endeavor. Secondly, to the many others who helped me over the years with their belief in me and their support of my goals.

Above all, I want to thank God. All my beliefs, opinions, and theories are based upon my belief that first, God created us, and second, He created us to be healthy.

Hosea 4:6 My people are destroyed for lack of knowledge.

Jesus said in John 10:10 "The thief cometh not, but for to steal, and to kill, and to destroy: I am come that they might have life, and that they might have *it* more abundantly." Being sick is not living an abundant life. I believe God gave us everything right here on earth that we need to stay healthy.

INTRODUCTION

I have been a naturopathic doctor for over fifteen years. My primary focus has always been identifying toxins in the body and eliminating them through the use of homeopathy and herbs.

I had asthma, skin problems, and allergies as a child. Some children seem to grow out of childhood health problems, but mine actually got worse as I grew older. I was the only child out of four in our family to have such severe health issues. My parents owned a health food store, so I had access to many alternative health methods and supplements. In spite of these supplements, nothing ever seemed to help. Unfortunately, much of the time, these alternative health methods only treat the symptoms. Most are just a healthier forms of treatment from traditional medicines but with fewer side effects.

I never bought into the idea that I was just born with asthma and eczema because I didn't have them as a baby. It took me years to realize that my health problems were the result of toxins in my body. In my teen years, I thought if I could just exercise enough I could stay healthy and my diet did not matter. Exercise did help, but my health steadily declined.

In my junior year of college, I became very sick and lost about thirty-five pounds. My normal weight was about 165, and this sudden, mysterious drop to 130 made me look and feel awful. I was brought up to rely on alternative health treatments, but nothing I tried was working. I decided at that point to go see a medical doctor. My parents were not supportive of this, and my mother even said, "Go right ahead, but they won't find anything." She was right! The young intern who saw me took a urine sample, but then dismissed me saying, "There's nothing wrong. You're fine!" I have never gone back to a medical doctor since. I recovered, but never really felt quite right again for many years. In addition to regular exercise, I also tried to eat better, which only slightly helped.

As my quest for health continued into my early thirties, I was tested on an EAV machine.[1] I immediately knew that this machine had the potential to finally give me the answers to my health issues. I became so excited about the possibilities of this new technology, that I became a naturopathic doctor. I purchased an EAV machine for myself, and began delving into learning as much as possible. EAV stands for electro acupuncture according to Voll. Dr. Voll was a German medical doctor who studied Chinese acupuncture in the 1950s and discovered there was an electrical current coming from each acupuncture point on the body.

Dr. Voll then went on to develop a machine that could measure that electrical current from an acupuncture point using a probe. A healthy human body has about nine micro amps of electricity. The machine measures if there is more or less than that coming from different acupuncture points that lead to various organs in the body. As technology progressed, a computer program was developed that stored the electrical frequencies of various toxins. The computer program also stored the electrical frequencies of various herbs, foods, and nutrients. Using the probe, one would touch an acupuncture point on the body and get a reading on the electrical flow coming from that point. If the reading was not normal, one can then test for toxins or nutritional deficiencies.

It sounds simple, but learning to use the EAV machine accurately takes many years of practice to become proficient. The EAV requires attention to detail in order to ensure accurate readings. There is an art to its use; to maintain consistency, there has to be a rigorous system of cross-checking the results. My incentive for becoming a naturopathic doctor and continuing in my quest for knowledge was that I desperately wanted to be well. With my many health problems, I believed that if I could get well, I could then help others to get well, too. By learning to diagnose toxins, followed by taking the correct homeopathics, herbs, and nutrition, I did eventually alleviate all of my health issues.

Through my search, I also have discovered there is often a spiritual aspect to disease. I refer you to a landmark book on this subject: *A More Excellent Way: A Teaching on the Spiritual Roots of Disease*, by Henry W. Wright. This book explains, in detail, how spiritual issues in our lives can, and do, affect us physically.

This twenty-year path I took to research and learn was a difficult one, but worth the investment. I'm writing this book to share hope. So many people are told to "grow old gracefully," and just accept their aches and pains because they are growing older. Age, by itself, is not a good enough reason to have pain. If you believe, like I do, that you can be healthy again, then keep reading, and let me show you how to experience that. Let's focus on becoming healthy.

OF COURSE YOU HAVE TOXINS!

I divide toxins into two groups: organic and inorganic. Within each group there are five categories. The organic category contains toxins one would be more likely to come into contact with by being outdoors. Examples would be working with soil, such as farming or gardening, swimming in a lake, river, or ocean, or just being in contact with other people or animals.

The inorganic category lists toxins one might come into contact with by visiting a medical doctor or dentist. Examples might be having X-rays or taking over the counter and/or prescription medications. Other possibilities may include working in a power or chemical plant, use of cell phones, spraying pesticides on one's lawn or garden, working with cleaning solvents, or wearing cosmetics. We will regularly come into contact with toxins throughout our lifetime. Toxins are just a reality in our environment.

Most of the focus in alternative health seems to be on inorganic toxins. The concerns are with mercury in fish, radiation from power plants, and pesticides in the air and food. While these are legitimate concerns, I have found that the majority of toxins in people are organic. I do find inorganic toxins, but usually at very low levels. In my estimation, 75% of the toxins in the average person are organic and the remaining 25% inorganic. Many times, people react with shock and surprise at the numerous toxins I discover in their body. Some react with disbelief, while others seem to feel hopeless. In America today, we have better hygiene than previous generations, as well as a better standard of living with running water and modern sewage systems, so we believe that toxins are not a problem. But stop for a minute and think about that - How many people actually stop and wash their hands after using a public restroom? How many pet owners wash their hands after playing with their pets? Have you ever been bitten by a mosquito-or any other type of insect? Animals and insects still pass toxins to humans even though we improved our standard of living.

ORGANIC	INORGANIC
Parasites	Chemicals
Bacteria	Medications
Fungi	Vaccines
Viruses	Heavy Metals
Venoms	Radiation

Just a few years ago, I met with a patient from Nebraska who traveled to a southern state and returned with health problems. She visited her doctor with a suspicion she had picked up parasites during her travels. The doctor told her, "There are no such thing as parasites in humans in this day and age." She then informed the doctor that she had seen them in her stool, and only then did he start to believe her. In my opinion, everyone, especially medical professionals, needs to have a much better understanding of the nature of toxins in our environment.

I am writing this book not only to bring awareness of the existence of toxins in our environment which can affect our bodies, but also to outline a process of elimination for better health. The good news is that you can rid the body of all of these toxins through the proper use of homeopathy, herbs, and nutrition.

TOXINS

tox·in (tăk-sən) **n.** [L. toxicum, poison]. A poisonous substance, especially a protein, that is produced by living cells or organisms and is capable of causing disease when introduced into the body tissues by interacting with biological macromolecules such as enzymes or cellular receptors.

The American Heritage Dictionary of the English Language, Fourth Edition, Houghton Mifflin Company, 2006.

ORGANIC TOXINS

OF COURSE YOU HAVE PARASITES!

The first question people have when I tell them they have parasites is, "How did I get them? The answer is they are all around us. Parasites can come from insect bites, family pets, undercooked food, contaminated drinking water, walking barefoot on contaminated soil, swimming in rivers, lakes, oceans, or breathing in contaminated soil in a dry, windy climate. Parasites are transmitted from animals to humans, from our environment to humans, and also from human to human.

Parasites are sensitive to the gravitational pull of the moon. As a result, they are more active at night and during a full moon. Many patients report that their symptoms appear worse in the evening hours and during a full moon. After years of finding parasites and studying them, I believe that many symptoms people experience could be from parasites.

Through my extensive research, I classify parasites into five categories. First, there are roundworms or nematodes such as pinworms, hookworms, threadworms, and whipworms. These are all common types of roundworms and most people have heard of them. Next, there are tapeworms or cestodes, which are also very common and well known. These parasites are easy to eliminate from the body by taking the proper herbs or medication.[2]

The next category is flukes or trematodes. Also called flatworms, these are the most common parasites I find. It is commonly thought that this type of parasite is only found in third-world countries. Since almost everyone I test shows up as having trematodes, I conclude they are not limited to third-world countries. These parasites are also the most difficult to eliminate. Even with the right herbal combination or medication, they take a little bit longer to rid from the body.

The next two categories are microscopic parasites: Filarial worms (microscopic roundworms) and Protozoa or Amoeba parasites. Usually the microscopic parasites are picked up from contaminated water or insect bites, like mosquitoes.

Possible parasite symptoms are to numerous to list because they can go just about anywhere in the body, especially the microscopic ones. In my experience, the most common symptoms are related to the intestines.

I know with myself, after eliminating my own parasites, my mind seemed clearer. It was like a fog had been lifted from my brain, and I could definitely think more clearly. Concentrating on things was no longer a chore. I also noticed fewer intestinal problems. Many patients have asked me why traditional doctors do not find parasites. I believe it has to do with their testing methods. I only know that I find them using my EAV machine. Plus it makes sense to me that if animals suffer from them, then certainly humans can as well. In later chapters, I will explain how to rid the body of parasites through safe and easy methods.

BACTERIA, FUNGI, AND VIRUSES

I like to put bacteria, fungi and viruses into the same category because they have similar characteristics. They can be transmitted to humans much the same way parasites are. They are transmitted through contact with soil, other people, animals, contaminated food or water or insect bites. Considering all the insect bites one receives throughout a lifetime, it is easy to imagine all of the possible toxins transmitted.

I consistently find bacteria, fungus, and virus toxins at either chronic or acute levels in my patients. Chronic means the toxins are more dormant, while acute means more active. Acute levels generally produce more symptoms. Unfortunately, traditional medicines such as antibiotics, do not eliminate the full spectrum of bacteria. Traditional doctors may have treatments for fungi and viruses, but generally not cures, which is why I still find them in my testing.

Another possible source for fungi is antibiotics because they are made from fungi, like penicillin. This is an effective treatment for the immediate symptoms, but for the overall health of the body, this is inefficient. Using one toxin to eliminate another is not efficient because it has introduced a new toxin into the body that now must be eliminated for optimal health.

Something that concerns me is when sickness is attributed to a single parasite, such as malaria, or a single bacterium, such as Lyme. The implication is that the person needs just one toxin removed from the body to regain optimum health. The problem with this assumption is that in most cases, it is not true. I have never tested anyone who had just one parasite, or just one bacterium. Since most people host a multitude of toxins and parasites in their bodies, it is best to take one remedy to eliminate an entire toxin category, or an entire spectrum of parasites.

Neurotransmitters

About a year ago I listened to a doctor who is considered to be an expert on neurotransmitters being interviewed on a Christian talk show. As a result, I started testing my patients for neurotransmitter deficiencies, and I found that many people are lacking in at least one.

Often I find that people are lacking one or more of these four neurotransmitters: serotonin, tryptophan, GABA, and dopamine. Most are lacking either tryptophan or serotonin. For humans, tryptophan is an essential amino acid. This means our bodies cannot synthesize or create it, therefore we must receive it from our diet. Tryptophan is a precursor for serotonin, and its principal function is to work as a building block in protein biosynthesis.

Tryptophan is known as a sleep aid, which is probably due to its ability to increase serotonin levels in the brain. Serotonin is responsible for aiding memory function, leveling emotions, and aiding sleep, appetite, and temperature regulation. Another neurotransmitter, dopamine, also has many functions in the brain. Dopamine is responsible for voluntary movement, cognition, motivation, and pleasure. Dopamine is also associated with addictions and love.

GABA is the abbreviation for Gamma-aminobutyric acid and is the primary inhibitory neurotransmitter in the central nervous system, which blocks the transmission of an impulse from one cell to another. This decreases the neuron activity and prevents them from over-firing. This activity prevents anxiety and stress related messages from reaching the motor centers of the brain.[3]

Not long after I started testing for neurotransmitter deficiencies, I started to see a correlation between what neurotransmitter a person was lacking and what bacteria, fungi or viruses they had. For instance, individuals who tested positive for the bacteria which causes Lyme disease, borrelia burgdorferi [4], also tested as lacking tryptophan. My theory is that people first pick up the bacteria, fungus or virus, which then causes a corresponding neurotransmitter deficiency. I know with myself, I was lacking in GABA until I completed my herbal detoxification regimen.

I have also tested Bach Flower remedies and found that each one is high in a particular neurotransmitter. If someone tests as needing one particular Bach Flower remedy, then they are probably lacking in the neurotransmitter that Bach Flower remedy happens to be high in.

What I have found is that if a person eliminates most or all of the toxins in his or her body, then they are no longer lacking in any neurotransmitters. The body is able to utilize the nutrients from food to produce the proper levels of neurotransmitters needed for optimum health.

AUTISM:
THE LEPTOSPIROSIS
AND SYNTHETIC
ESTROGEN CONNECTION

Autism is a developmental disorder of the central nervous system which usually manifests before the age of three. There is no blood test or biological marker for autism, so it is diagnosed using specific criteria for testing social interaction skills, communication skills, and restricted and repetitive behaviors. Reported cases of autism spectrum disorders have increased greatly since the 1990s. Some estimates of reported cases are as high as one in every 150 children (Centers for Disease Control), while others are as low as one out of every 1000 (National Institute of Mental Health). There are many theories as to the specific cause or causes of autism, but they are as of yet unproven. The causes, symptoms, and treatments all seem to be controversial.[5]

I have tested numerous children with autism and have found five distinct and compelling similarities in all cases. First, a primary toxin always present, without exception, is a type of bacterium called leptospirosis. Leptospirosis is caused by a spirochaete bacterium called leptospira. Other examples of sprochaetal bacteria would be borrelia burgdorferi, which causes Lyme disease, and treponema pallidum, which causes syphilis. I am not sure why this connection has gone unnoticed in the study and treatment of autism, but I do know that antibiotics seem to be ineffective against any sprochaetal bacteria. There is a foundation (www.lymeinducedautism.com) looking into a possible Lyme/autism connection, although my research does not support this. The only connection I have found is that some patients with autism have both the Leptospirosis and Lyme bacteria present.

In addition to acute levels of leptospirosis, children with autism also have high levels of fungi and protozoa parasites. They are also lacking in the neurotransmitter serotonin. Curiously, their tests also reveal the presence of synthetic estrogen. The question is, where did the synthetic estrogen come from? Possible sources include birth control pills or hormones in the food supply. Synthetic estrogen has even been found in plastic water and soda bottles.

Out of the five compelling similarities I have mentioned, the leptospirosis bacterium, the protozoa parasites, and the synthetic estrogen are the only toxins that current researchers have not identified as possible contributors to autism. Since many people test positive for protozoa parasites, they are less likely a significant factor than the leptospirosis bacterium and the synthetic estrogen. I am not sure at this point the role synthetic estrogen plays in contributing to autism. Researchers are already aware that children with autism have high levels of fungi and are lacking in serotonin. I look forward to more research being devoted to leptospirosis and synthetic estrogen as possible culprits. The good news is I have developed effective herbal remedies which in my testing show the elimination of these toxins.

VENOMS

Last from the organic group are venoms. Venoms are comprised of enzymes and other proteins that are sometimes hemotoxic,[6] meaning they destroy red blood cells, disrupting blood clotting and causing organ or tissue damage. Some venoms are neurotoxic,[6] meaning they affect the nervous system by disrupting or damaging neurons. Occasionally, venoms are both hemotoxic and neurotoxic. Again, the correct herbal combinations can eliminate these toxins.

The Stories of Michael and Robert

Michael and Robert are both successful Oregon businessmen. Each came to me with serious health problems resulting from venoms.

Michael's foot was badly swollen, discolored, and painful. He was symptomatic for five weeks and nothing he tried was helping. Testing his blood, I found a high level of spider venom. After just one day of taking my remedies he experienced relief. Within a few days his foot was back to normal.

Robert had a terrible rash all over his body and was miserable because it was itching so badly. After identifying the culprit as spider venom, I started him on a course of treatment. His itching subsided within hours of taking my herbal remedies, and within a couple of weeks the rash was almost completely gone.

Both Michael and Robert were anxious for relief, not only because they were suffering, but also because they are both in the business of selling nutritional products. They were concerned their maladies would reflect negatively on their credibility with customers.

INORGANIC TOXINS

CHEMICALS

Technically, there is not much difference between chemicals and heavy metals. Many chemicals have heavy metal compounds in them. In fact, the lines separating my five categories of inorganic toxins are subtle. When thinking of chemicals, pesticides often come to mind. Many pesticides used in the past were nothing more than heavy metals such as arsenic and mercury.[7] Many traditional medicines contain trace amounts of heavy metals. Amalgam fillings used by dentists for 150 years contain mercury, silver, as well as other heavy metals. Small amounts of heavy metals and even radiation can sometimes be found in vaccines. A few years ago, Thimerosal was in the news due to its use in vaccines. A mercury-based preservative chosen for its bacteriostatic properties, it is now being phased out due to serious health risks.

Three methods are used in the attenuation, or weakening, of a bacteria or virus used in a vaccine: high heat, chemicals, and radiation. The main reason I separate vaccines from other medications is because of the use of rDNA,[8] or recombinant DNA. This process allows the vaccine to combine with human DNA making it more difficult to eliminate than any other toxin. A great resource concerning the dangers of vaccines is the book, *A Shot in the Dark: Why the P in the DPT Vaccination May Be Hazardous to Your Child's Health*, by Harris L. Coulter and Barbara Loe Fisher.

Some heavy metals, such as uranium, are radioactive. The toxic affects on the body are similar for heavy metals and radiation. In the human body, when free radicals react with heavy metals or radiation, the number of free radical molecules increases. A free radical is an atom or molecule with an unpaired electron. This causes a chain reaction with harmful effects. An example would be the molecules which make up water, or H_2O. This means there are two hydrogen molecules and one oxygen molecule. When radiation invades the body, it changes the molecular structure of water from H_2O to HO. As a result, the HO has become a free radical spinning around causing damage to cells. Since there is a loose, unpaired electron, the HO looks for another hydrogen atom to steal from another molecule. Once the HO finds and steals that hydrogen atom, the process begins once again—the new HO starts damaging cells, which then does likewise to another.[9]

The Story of Dan

When I first met Dan, he was a forty year old farmer who had just been diagnosed with a sudden onset of rheumatoid arthritis. He walked slowly into my office, each step showing obvious pain. During testing, I identified an acute level of tetanus vaccine. He explained he recently received a new shot just a few weeks earlier due to a minor accident on the farm.

I recommended a homeopathic remedy to help remove the vaccine residue. After just a few days, his wife called to tell me Dan was feeling much better and was able to move without pain. Today Dan is still farming without any symptoms of rheumatoid arthritis.

FINAL THOUGHTS ON TOXINS

We eat, drink, touch, and even breathe toxins daily—they are everywhere, and we are in constant contact with them. Bacteria, parasites, molds, and pollens have been around for centuries…it is not realistic to attempt to avoid them altogether. Good hygiene practices are a wise preventative measure, although my testing of soaps indicates that most lack an ability to destroy bacteria and viruses. The major benefit comes from the simple action of rinsing the germs off the body with a surfactant and water. Also, many people use mosquito repellants but still get bitten, so the use of repellants as a preventative is not 100% reliable.

In my opinion, our focus should be on prevention, not avoidance. Supplementing your diet with the right herbs and nutrition gives the best protection against invading toxins by supplying all the necessary enzymes and cofactors. These nutrients destroy the toxins before symptoms manifest. If we ingest the proper nutrition daily, we will protect ourselves from becoming sick. With knowledge, we can escape the fear of toxins.

The following chapters will explain how the proper remedies can give the best defense and prevention against toxins. I will be covering homeopathy and herbs, why they work, and which are most more efficient.

REMEDIES

rem·e·dy (rem'i-dē) **n.** [L. remedium, medicine]. To cure or relieve a disease. Any medicine, treatment, or therapy that cures, heals, or relieves a disease or bodily disorder or tends to restore health. A means of putting something right or getting rid of something undesirable.

The American Heritage Stedman's Medical Dictionary, Houghton Mifflin Company, 2002.

HOMEOPATHY

The theory and practice of homeopathy is strange to those of us who are accustomed to conventional Western medicine. The word homeopathy comes from the Greek words homoios (similar) and pathos (suffering or disease). Literally, it means "like with like" or the "same disease treats the same disease." Homeopathy is designed to assist the body to heal itself. In the late 1700's, homeopathy emerged as a highly systematic healing art due to the efforts of a German physician and chemist, Dr. Samuel Hahnemann.

Dr. Hahnemann revealed that substances that cause a disease, or particular set of symptoms, could also relieve the disease if it was diluted in doses so minute that no molecules of the original substance remained, only the electrical frequency. Hahnemann coined the phrase "let like cure like" to describe his discovery that substances in small doses stimulate the body to conquer toxins that cause illness in higher amounts. This principle is most commonly known as the Law of Similars.

There are three categories in homeopathy: nosodes, isodes, and sarcodes.[10] Nosodes are remedies created from disease-causing organisms. To make a homeopathic nosode, a sample of a disease-causing organism is diluted to a homeopathic level. This is accomplished by placing the organism into a mixture of distilled water and alcohol then vigorously shaking the solution, also called succussion. This dilution process is continued until the desire potency level is achieved. Due to the toxicity of the original disease-causing specimen used for the creation of the nosode, the dilution should continue unti; all that remains is the electrical imprint of the organism in the nosode.

Any homeopathic diluted to this level is considered high potency. The more a homeopathic is diluted, the stronger it becomes because of its transition to an electrical frequency. The remedy at this point is a liquid formula containing water, alcohol, and an electrical frequency. By using this process, Dr. Hahnemann determined the correct potency necessary to create a sustained healing response, although the resulting remedy is considered fragile. For instance, a magnet or an electrical appliance can negatively impact its effectiveness.

When taking a high potency homeopathic remedy containing an electrical imprint, the potency needs to be the resonating frequency of the toxin. In physics, resonance is the tendency of an object to oscillate or vibrate at maximum amplitude at a certain frequency.[11] Atoms and molecules have special resonant frequencies that will only be excited by energies of precise vibratory characteristics. Resonance is the principle behind the imaging systems of EMR and MRI scanning machines. For instance, the singer who is able to shatter a wine glass by delivering a high amplitude note does so by singing in the precise resonant frequency of the glass.[12] In homeopathy, when a substance is potentized and taken as a remedy, it acts like a pole of one magnet pushing against another magnetic pole of like charge. Hence, the disease entity is essentially excreted from the body. As a result, the disease process is eradicated and consequently, so is the root cause of the disease.

A disadvantage to the homeopathic nosode approach is the possibility of a healing crisis, commonly referred to as a Herxheimer Reaction.[13] This is a short-term immune system reaction to the toxins which are released when large amounts of pathogens are being destroyed and the body does not eliminate these endotoxins quickly enough.[14] Endotoxins are toxins released from within a pathogen as they are eliminated. The Herxheimer Reaction is a normal and even healthy reaction which indicates parasites, bacteria, fungi, viruses, or other pathogens are being detoxified.

As the body detoxifies, it is not uncommon to experience cold or flu-like symptoms for a few days. These symptoms could include: headaches, joint and muscle pain, sore throat, general lethargy, sweating, chills, sinus congestion, skin eruptions, nausea, diarrhea, or other symptoms. These occur when the body is detoxifying and the released endotoxins either exacerbate the symptoms being treated or create their own symptoms.

It is important to note that worsening symptoms do not indicate failure of the treatment; in fact, just the opposite. The biggest problem with the Herxheimer Reaction is that people often completely stop taking the supplement or medication. A better course of action would be to temporarily discontinue the treatment until symptoms subside, then slowly resume the regimen again.

Isodes are the next category in homeopathy. An isode is a remedy created from anything that is not a disease-causing organism. Most isode formulas are meant to only treat the symptoms. They can be low potency or high potency depending on the toxicity of the components used. If one takes something that causes symptoms in a non-diluted form, then in a diluted form it should treat those same symptoms. An example would be quinine. Quinine is made from the bark of the South American cinchona tree and has been used for years to treat malaria.[15]

Quinine can be toxic in its non-diluted form and cause some of the same symptoms as malaria. Malaria is a protozoa parasite that is usually transmitted by mosquitoes. The symptoms of malaria include high fever, vomiting, cramping, and diarrhea. The body wants to purge the parasite any way it can. The body is thrown into an acute condition where it tries to combat the parasite. Many people who die from malaria actually die from dehydration.

Quinine, in a diluted homeopathic form, stops the acute symptoms, but really does not kill the malaria parasite. It is more of a treatment than a cure. There is an obvious advantage to this because a life can be saved. One still has malaria, but the acute symptoms are gone and now the malaria is more of a chronic condition.

The last category of homeopathy is sarcodes. Sarcodes are homeopathic glandular extracts, such as raw adrenal or raw thyroid. Their purpose is in supporting endocrine glands. Most glandular supplements are in tablet or capsule form. The advantage of a homeopathic is it bypasses digestion to reach the targeted organ. Most people with compromised endocrine glands also have digestive problems.

HERBS AND METABOLIC ENZYMES

Many people assume that herbs work in the same way as traditional medication by simply killing off the disease-causing organism. I do not believe this to be the case. Herbs break down into enzymes and nutrients, which are referred to as cofactors. What is different about the way herbs work is their combination of enzymes and cofactors. My theory is that together these enzymes and their cofactors digest the parasites. This explains why many times people do not experience a healing crisis while detoxifying with herbs.

An enzyme is a catalyst which speeds up reactions within living organisms. All enzymes are catalysts, but not all catalysts are enzymes. Some people are familiar with enzymes, such as digestive enzymes, but very few know about metabolic enzymes. Metabolic enzymes are defined as any enzyme produced within the body that is not utilized for digestion. Metabolic enzymes, especially in humans, speed up reactions within cells, tissues, and organs. These reactions slow down aging in cells, and help regulate cellular processes such as mitosis and cell respiration. As with all enzymes, metabolic enzymes require vitamins, minerals, and other cofactors to work properly.[16]

A cofactor is a non-protein chemical compound that is tightly bound to an enzyme as a catalyst and assists in biochemical transformations. In other words, it speeds up the reaction rate an enzyme has with food or toxins. Cofactors allow metabolic enzymes to digest toxins they could never digest on their own. I cannot over-emphasize the importance of cofactors to the proper function of enzymes. Minerals and amino acids are common cofactors. Vitamins are usually considered coenzymes. Rather than directly contributing to the catalytic ability of an enzyme, coenzymes participate with the enzyme in the catalytic reaction. Often this distinction is no longer made, and coenzymes are used in the broader sense as cofactors.[17]

I believe these metabolic enzymes and cofactors will digest most, if not all toxins in the body, even chemicals and other non-living organisms. Our bodies produce both digestive and metabolic enzymes. Most foods that we eat like fruits, vegetables, meats, and dairy contain enzymes which aide in digestion as well. We also need help with digesting toxins, but the problem is that the metabolic enzymes which are capable of this, are rare in foods that we normally eat. We also tend to heat up our food before eating it much of the time, which destroys these critical enzymes. Often the foods which contain these metabolic enzymes do not contain the cofactors necessary for the enzymes to work properly. Therefore, the best source for these metabolic enzymes and their cofactors is herbs. Raw herbs, like Echinacea, contain these metabolic enzymes and the proper cofactors. The key is to find the herbs which contain the proper levels of enzymes and cofactors necessary to eliminate toxins.

These metabolic enzymes are also found naturally in bacteria and fungi. Bacteria contain some of them, but fungi actually contain more. The right combination of fungi which contain enough of a variety of metabolic enzymes can kill off, or digest, a broad spectrum of bacteria. The only problem with this approach is that fungi do not naturally contain enough of a variety of metabolic enzymes to kill off the entire spectrum of bacteria. Fungi and bacteria also do not contain any cofactors, which would explain why antibiotics do not work against fungi and viruses. Viruses, by the way, do not contain any metabolic enzymes. People also assume herbs will destroy the good bacteria, or gut flora, in our digestive tract like antibiotics do. Metabolic enzymes do not kill off, or digest, our good bacteria.

Diseases not directly linked to a nutritional deficiency could be due to an enzyme imbalance. If nutritional needs have been met, yet a person is sick, an enzyme imbalance or deficiency could be the culprit.[18] Many diseases are known to be due to a deficiency of a single enzyme. An example would be carbohydrate-deficient glycoprotein syndrome (CDGS), which is a deficiency in the metabolic enzyme phosphomannose isomerase (PMI). The disorder is caused by mutations in the PMI1 gene.[19]

The higher your metabolic enzyme production and intake, the greater your ability to cleanse, heal, and regenerate. Another question that is asked of me is, "Do our bodies produce enough metabolic enzymes?" The answer is no. The toxin exposure occurring environmentally creates the necessity of supplemental metabolic enzymes.

A great resource for finding what kinds of nutrients are in herbs is the book, *Nutritional Herbology: A Reference Guide to Herbs*, by Mark Peterson. The author is a research chemist who specializes in herbal chemistry. He tested many herbs in a laboratory and wrote this comprehensive encyclopedia of herbs, including a scientific analysis of their nutrients.

THE IMPORTANCE OF COFACTORS

Everyone has heard of nutrients such as vitamins, minerals, amino acids, and enzymes, but few have heard of other nutrients called phenolics. Some examples of phenolics are valeric acid, urushiol, gallic acid, and vanillin. Phenolics are a class of organic chemical compounds found in many foods that we eat. The problem is that they often occur naturally in foods at very low levels, while we need higher levels of certain ones for optimum health.

Phenolics often referred to as antioxidants, are considered to be a type of phytonutrient, or secondary metabolite. They are also sometimes referred to as phytochemicals.[20] Secondary metabolites are organic compounds which are not directly essential for sustaining life, but are essential for maintaining good health. Phenolics come from either plant or animal sources. They promote the function of the immune system to fight off toxins such as bacteria and viruses, plus they reduce inflammation.

There seems to be an attitude in Western society that we should only take the minimum amount of vitamins and supplemental nutrients. I understand the need for balance and safety, but our bodies need higher levels of certain nutrition. The RDA, or Recommended Daily Allowance, which is now called the RDI, or Reference Daily Intake, is based upon the minimum our bodies need for survival, not necessarily what our bodies need for optimum health. Currently the United States Department of Agriculture sets these guidelines. Through my testing, I have found that all adults need about the same amount, though this may vary slightly according to size and physical activity. I have also found that children only need about half the amount of adults.

Many people assume that all they need to do to reach the proper dosage of these phytonutrients is to eat enough fruits and vegetables each day, but this does not even supply half of the dosage of these nutrients that we need daily. Therefore, it becomes necessary to get them from other sources. In my opinion, herbs are the best choice for the proper intake of these nutrients. Certain herbs contain high enough levels of all the metabolic enzymes, vitamins, minerals, trace elements, amino acids and phytonutrients that we need each day to keep our bodies free of toxins. Even if a person has achieved high enough levels of vitamins, minerals, amino acids, and enzymes through diet and supplementation on a regular basis, it is still not enough to maximize health. One must also have enough of the other nutrients, such as certain phenolics, in order to experience optimum health. Remember, vitamins, minerals, amino acids, and enzymes are necessary for sustaining life, but phenolics are necessary for sustaining good health.

MIASMS

I would like to make a comment about congenital toxins. In homeopathy, the term for an inherited toxin is miasm.[21] Miasma, from the Greek, means stain. I do not agree with Samuel Hahnemann's theories on miasms. He asserted that the underlying root causes of all chronic diseases of mankind were three fundamental toxins: Sycosis, meaning Gonorrhea, Syphilis, and Psora.

When I test for toxins in the blood after a person has taken the initial 6–8 week prescribed dose of my remedy, what I find is what I have always assumed to be vaccine toxins. I am assuming these toxins are from vaccines, but there is a small chance they could possibly be toxins inherited from the parents. The same remedy would be used for each because both vaccines and inherited toxins would be attached to the DNA.[22]

It makes sense to me that if medications, such as Diethylstilbestrol (DES)—and Thalidomide, can cause birth defects, then vaccines, which are attached to the DNA, could also be passed congenitally. Thalidomide is a sedative that was given to pregnant women for morning sickness in the 1960s. Some babies died and others suffered from birth defects such as deafness, blindness, and disfigurement.[23]

In the 1940's, DES was prescribed for pregnant women to help prevent miscarriages. In 1971 it was found to be teratogenic, causing birth defects.[24] There have been some studies done on vaccines being possible teratogens. In particular, anthrax vaccines given to military personnel have been under study since the Gulf War.[25] Also, MMR vaccine studies have been done, but nothing conclusive has been proven.

ENDOCRINE GLANDS

The thyroid is the largest endocrine glands in the body. It controls how quickly the body burns energy. The thyroid produces hormones that regulate the growth and rate of function of many other systems in the body. The two principle hormones it produces are thyroxine (T4) and triiodothyronine (T3). The thyroid gland gets its name from the Greek word for shield. It is controlled by the hypothalamus and the pituitary, which along with the thyroid are often compromised by toxins. The pituitary gland is considered the master gland and secretes hormones that regulate homeostasis. The hypothalamus links the nervous system to the endocrine system through the pituitary gland.[26]

The pituitary gland is usually compromised by microscopic parasites, bacteria, fungi, and viruses. Other glands and organs can be affected by a variety of toxins. Once the majority of toxins are removed through the detoxification process, the thyroid is usually the only remaining gland with toxin issues. The good news is that once the remaining toxins are removed, and proper nutrition is taken, the thyroid gland is also able to recover.

THE SUCCESSFUL SOLUTION

Herbs

When I first began testing people years ago, I quickly found that almost everyone has parasites. As a result, I focused my research on parasites, and began looking for a good remedy to eliminate them. After an unsatisfactory search for an effective remedy, I decided to develop my own formula. Most of the remedies I found worked well for roundworms and tapeworms, but not for flatworms, or flukes, which are the most common.

I also had difficulty finding remedies that were effective against the microscopic parasites. I found that one not only needs the correct herbal combinations, but also the proper milligrams of those herbs. I tested many herbal remedies that had the correct ingredients, but not the proper milligrams of those herbs to work against the whole spectrum of parasites. I had a great advantage with my machine because I had access to a wide variety of frequencies of parasites, and the computer program also included the electrical frequencies of herbs that I could test against those parasite frequencies. I developed an herbal remedy that also included homeopathics and nutrition. Later, the FDA decided homeopathics could no longer be included with herb,s so my current formulas only contain herbs and nutrition. They work very effectively against the entire spectrum of parasites.

I have taken each individual herb used in my formulas and broken it down to identify its nutritional components. Each has varying degrees of vitamins, minerals, amino acids, enzymes and other components. Two herbs may have some of the same nutrients but at different levels. Further testing revealed what nutrients are necessary to eliminate each category of toxins. For example, one group of nutrients eliminates the entire spectrum of parasites, while another combination eliminates the entire spectrum of bacteria. These combinations include all the necessary metabolic enzymes and their cofactors in their correct amounts. In the beginning, my assumption was that the metabolic enzymes would need to be at higher levels than the cofactors, but this is not always the case.

As a result, a person needs to have the correct nutrients, but also have those nutrients at the proper levels, which is why many herbal remedies do not eliminate the entire spectrum of parasites and other toxins. Without the proper levels, or milligrams, the desired results will not be achieved. This would not pertain to herbs used in homeopathic combinations. As a result, homeopathic herbal combinations are not quite as efficient at treating the entire spectrum of toxins because they can't eliminate vaccine residue entirely.

I successfully double-checked my findings by testing just the nutrients found in the herbs against various toxins. The nutrients tested as eliminating the toxins by themselves without the whole herb being used, thus proving to me that it was the metabolic enzymes and their cofactors that actually did the work of eliminating the toxins.

Another important factor I have found that needs to be taken into consideration is which form of an herb is being utilized. For instance, Echinacea Angustifolia has many nutrients in it, i.e., metabolic enzymes and cofactors. On the other hand, Echinacea Purpurea only contains a few nutrients. Therefore, Echinacea Angustifolia is preferable to the Echinacea Purpurea for detoxifying. To be fair, there may be other benefits to Echinacea Purpurea that I am not aware of, but for the purpose of detoxification, Echinacea Angustifoila is more beneficial. The part of the herb being used can make a difference, too. Sometimes it is better to use the stalk rather than the root, while with a different herb, the opposite may be true.

Homeopathics

Over the course of many years, I became more and more frustrated with the homeopathics available on the market. I also found that most homeopathic and herbal remedies for toxins did not work. I tested many remedies against a vast array of toxins, but was severely disappointed. I felt the need to create remedies which would actually produce the desired results, so I formulated my own.

My first remedy was an herbal capsule called Miavax. I soon realized I needed a liquid homeopathic version for anyone who could not swallow capsules, so I developed PAR-X. Both of these original formulas were just for parasites. I later modified the Miavax formula so that it was able to eliminate all toxins.

The next homeopathic I developed was for eliminating bacteria, fungi and viruses. Most companies divide these into three separate formulas. I considered doing that, too, but found through my testing that it really wasn't necessary. I was able to create an herbal homeopathic formula that could treat all three toxins effectively, and I named this formula BFV-X.

I next developed a homeopathic for chemical toxins. I originally thought I would have to develop one for each individual category, but after testing, I found that CHEM-X successfully treated a wide range of chemical toxins. To remove venoms from the body, I created VENOM-X.

My wife Laura challenged me to create just one remedy which would eliminate all toxins. After extensive testing, I developed an herbal combination which in my opinion has all of the necessary metabolic enzymes and cofactors in it to treat all toxins. It also contains the proper milligrams of those herbs. It is an herbal liquid, I named DETOXED.

For those people who prefer capsules over liquids, I created an updated formula for Miavax, which is now an herbal capsule version of DETOXED. A person can take this formula every day to receive the proper levels of necessary nutrients for optimum health. However, I have learned from working with patients over the years that it is best to begin the detoxification program with the homeopathic formulas, as there is much less chance of a Herxheimer Reaction. So, I developed a homeopathic version of DETOXED called Compre-tox. After the initial detoxification phase using Compre-tox, it is then safe to remove the remaining toxins with stronger herbal combinations like Miavax or DETOXED.

I realize that people need to get the bulk of their vitamins, minerals, and amino acids from their diet, not supplements. This is because food contains digestive enzymes that help us assimilate these nutrients, and the supplements do not. Unfortunately, many people try to get the bulk of their vitamins and minerals from their supplements and use their diet to supply the rest. This is not the preferable approach.

I decided to experiment with adding certain foods to the diet in combination with the DETOXED remedy instead of more herbs. I found that by adding certain nuts and seeds to the diet, in combination with the herbs in the DETOXED remedy, it completed the necessary combination. This worked because the body needs certain digestive enzymes in order to effectively assimilate the nutrients in the herbs. I combined the oils from these nuts and seeds to make a new formula to be taken in combination with the DETOXED, named DETOXOIL.

When working with patients, I have found that after taking the remedies for 6–8 weeks the follow-up test reveals that all the previous toxins are gone except some of the vaccine residues. The focus from this point on is entirely upon removing the vaccine toxins.

My patients frequently ask, "When the vaccine residue is removed, will that negate the protection the vaccine was meant to give me?" My answer is, "Definitely not!" I couldn't remove the antibodies from someone even if I wanted to. Our bodies build antibodies to the bacteria or virus from the vaccine upon receiving the shot.

What is being removed is excess residue that can cause more harm than good if left in the body, yet the immunity remains. Some people are symptom free after two months, but for the majority of my patients, some symptoms remain until the vaccine residue is entirely eliminated.

SYMPTOM LIST

Here is a list of the symptoms which I have eliminated through herbal detoxification.

- Asthma
- Bloating
- Constipation
- Cramps
- Diarrhea
- Difficulty Concentrating
- Fatigue
- Fluid Retention
- Food Allergies
- Frequent Urination
- Gum Disorders
- Heartburn
- Insomnia
- Intestinal Gas
- Joint and Muscle Pain and Stiffness

- Memory Difficulties
- Numbness and Tingling in Extremities
- Pollen Allergies (Hay Fever)
- Rashes and other Skin Irritations
- Sinus Congestion and Sensitivity to Odors
- Watery Eyes

NUTRITION IN YOUR DIET

In the first few years of my practice, I found that most people are deficient in at least some nutrition. The average person is lacking in minerals more often than vitamins, so I assume the average diet generally supplies enough vitamins, but not enough minerals.

The main minerals the average person is deficient in are magnesium, potassium, sodium, and a few trace minerals. The number one mineral people are lacking is magnesium. Magnesium is considered an essential nutrient and is one of the most abundant minerals found in the body. It plays a significant role in converting carbohydrates, protein, and fat into energy. Magnesium is important for the electrical stability of the cells, as well as maintaining membrane integrity.

Magnesium is associated with the functions of muscle relaxation and constriction, in addition to nerve transmission and conduction. It also has the ability to regulate and maintain vascular tone in the body and, as a cofactor, is necessary in over 3,000 enzymatic processes in the body. Magnesium also appears to regulate the ability of calcium to enter into cells to switch on vital functions, such as the heartbeat. It is essential for the assimilation of calcium and therefore has an important function in maintaining bone integrity. Recent research has even shown that magnesium plays a key role in rebuilding the body both during and after any detoxification program. National dietary surveys reveal that the average U.S. diet supplies only about half of the RDA of magnesium.

I, myself, tested deficient in magnesium. I tried to keep up with my body's demand through supplementation, but was unable to do so. I was extremely frustrated as to why so many people, including myself, lacked magnesium. Through more analysis, I discovered the reason is because most foods contain digestive enzymes which help us assimilate nutrients, such as magnesium, more efficiently than supplements.

Our bodies assimilate nutrients more effectively from food than from supplements, even though a supplement may contain much higher milligrams of a particular nutrient. Most herbs that do contain digestive enzymes only supply them at very low levels. There are many digestive enzymes and each have a purpose. Some digestive enzymes are for helping us assimilate vitamins, minerals and amino acids from our food and others help our bodies assimilate phytonutrients. An example of one of the enzymes I have found responsible for helping our bodies use nutrients more efficiently is intrinsic factor.

Intrinsic factor is a glycoprotein produced by the parietal cells of the stomach. It is essential for the assimilation of vitamin B12. A lack of intrinsic factor can lead to pernicious anemia and vitamin B12 deficiency. Even people ingesting adequate amounts of B12, can still be deficient in it if they do not have enough intrinsic factor.[27] Most of the foods we typically eat contain only low levels of intrinsic factor. Notable exceptions are strawberries and cacao, which contain the highest concentration of intrinsic factor of any foods that I have tested.

I believe most people do not receive enough intrinsic factor on a daily basis. To ensure that our bodies produce enough intrinsic factor, a person needs to receive adequate amounts of amino acids from animal source protein. To ensure a complete supply, a person also needs to take adequate amounts from an outside source, such as foods that contain intrinsic factor like strawberries and cacao.

There are two key states to the body–alkaline or acidic. In some medical circles, it is believed that a body that is acidic is more prone to getting cancer, so it is better to attempt to have a more alkaline state to the body. There are many books and articles devoted to the influence of diet on alkalinity. One benefit of an alkaline system is that it makes the body an unfavorable environment for parasites, bacteria, fungi, and viruses, which should result in fewer colds and flus. Parasites seem to thrive in a more acidic environment.

My testing has shown me that certain phenolics contribute to keeping our bodies alkaline. I have found the highest concentration of phenolics in beef, but they are also at high levels in dairy and eggs. Phenolics are also found in fruits and vegetables, but typically in smaller amounts. However, even with a high protein diet, certain oils from nuts and seeds along with the correct herbal combination are needed at the proper milligrams to complete the needed supplementation.

Also, our endocrine system needs some fat in order to function properly. I used to take raw glandular supplements, but have never needed them since changing my diet. I also maintain a normal cholesterol level. Many people who try the Atkin's diet only increase their protein levels. They are afraid of increasing their fat intake because of the current information on too much fat leading to health problems. They also tend not to increase their water intake. The result of not enough fat and water in the diet is constipation. Our bodies need water each day, but the amount varies depending on the person's size and physical activity.

A good rule to follow is to take half of your body weight and drink that number in ounces. For example, if a person weighs 150 lbs., the number of ounces of water consumed each day should be at least 75. On average, most people should drink at least 3 liters of water a day, or almost one gallon. Making sure one eats enough fat in the diet will also help prevent constipation.

Food Allergies

It is common knowledge that many people have allergies to foods such as peanuts. I have found that peanuts, strawberries, and sesame seeds contain some of the same digestive enzymes. These enzymes are typically found in lower amounts in many other foods. Since higher levels of these enzymes seem to be somewhat rare, I have to wonder if the reason people react to them is because the enzymes are digesting toxins. The reactions could possibly be similar to a Herxheimer Reaction. Their bodies might not be used to having higher levels of those enzymes on a regular basis and it would make sense that they might experience the same reaction as someone detoxifying for the first time.

I know many people feel that since they have allergies to certain foods, that they will never be able to eat those foods again. When I was a child, tests from the doctor showed that I had many food allergies. I am now able to eat whatever I want without any side affects. My opinion is that toxins in the body cause reactions not only to foods, but also pollens. I also had many pollen allergies that aggravated my asthma condition, but these have all disappeared since I eliminated the toxins in my body.

The Importance of Digestive Enzymes

Most people probably view food the way I used to. They assume that when they are experiencing hunger cravings, all they need to do is eat any food they want as long as it fills the stomach until a satisfied feeling is achieved; once the stomach feels full, this means they have done their job of keeping the body satisfied.

This is a mistake because our body is not only telling us that it needs food, but also that it is craving, or needs, certain nutrients. The problem is finding exactly what nutrients are needed, at what levels they are needed, and which foods to eat to satisfy the body's needs.

Stress is usually the trigger for cravings that occur between meals. Typically, the stress is either physical or emotional. Some examples of physical stress would be shivering when we feel cold, or being overly tired. An example of emotional stress would be feeling upset or nervous about someone or something. Most people experience an increase in these stresses as they grow older and the responsibilities of life change. If we feed our bodies what they are really craving, then we won't be continually craving food throughout each day. What determines how soon we feel hungry again after a meal is how well we supplied our body with the nutrients it needed with the previous meal. Supplying these necessary nutrients on a regular basis will help our body handle stress better, plus eliminate much of the cravings in between regular meals.

I know for myself, for years I would eat breakfast and then a few hours later I was hungry again. I remember the feeling that I was craving something, but I didn't know what. I usually ended up eating too much of several things. It took the edge off, because it satisfied my hunger, but I still felt like something was missing.

This is a common vicious cycle that people experience every day across the world. In my opinion, what is missing is digestive enzymes. We do ingest many digestive enzymes from various foods, but typically not at high enough levels. When we do ingest enzymes at high enough levels, then our bodies function much more efficiently. Our blood sugar is more easily regulated by the pancreas, and we do not experience all of the cravings between meals.

ATHLETIC PERFORMANCE

In my opinion, most people who do not exercise probably do not want to because they do not feel good enough to do it. They reach an age in their late 30's or early 40's when they start feeling aches and pains throughout their body so they no longer feel like exercising. In my opinion, this is due to a build up of toxins in their body. Once the toxins are eliminated, the desire to exercise is allowed to return because they no longer feel pain and stiffness all the time. All the organs can function as they should and constant fatigue is no longer an issue. Eliminating toxins may also help protect the body from exercise injuries such as muscle pulls and sprains.

Of course, part of this process is mentally starting a new habit. Along with any exercise program, though, a person needs to eat a proper diet. The success of any exercise or weight loss program is determined by what happens in the kitchen, not just the gym. We need protein and enough proper nutrients for muscle repair so that we continue to build up the body instead of tearing it down.

Getting enough nutrients in to the body is often the last thing people consider when starting an exercise program. They only seem to be interested in the final outcome from the actual exercising, like looking and feeling better. In my opinion, to be truly healthy, one also needs to consider nutrition and make that as much of a priority as the exercising.

I have often wondered why many other animal species are so much stronger than humans. Animals such as cattle, horses, apes, and bears all seem to grow stronger from their diet, not necessarily just the work their muscles do. Of course they grow stronger as they exercise, but they are genetically programmed to be stronger than humans even without exercising. Just from eating their normal diets they grow to be many times stronger than the strongest human. A human has to exercise in order to become very strong. Many other species are able to naturally manufacture sufficient amounts of the amino acids necessary for good health from plant source foods, which the human body seems to lack the ability to accomplish.

Our bodies require twenty different amino acids, of which eight or nine are generally regarded as essential because they cannot be produced, synthesized, or stored by the body. Non-essential amino acids are still very important and our bodies are able to synthesize them in sufficient amounts to meet the demands for growth and tissue repair.[28]

For humans, all essential amino acids may be obtained from plant sources, but it is much more difficult to obtain the levels our bodies require for optimum health using this approach. Being able to make sufficient protein from plant source foods may be considered an advantage that these other species have over us as far as obtaining strength, and in many cases, size, but we have nutritional requirements for brain function that they do not require.[29]

I would not want to suggest that we could become as strong as other species by improving our diet, but I do believe that we can become stronger than we currently are by making sure we receive sufficient amounts of nutrients and enzymes. This would serve a dual purpose; it would keep our bodies free of toxins, and it would also supply the nutrition needed for optimum health. As humans, we are limited as to how strong we can become. We will never reach the strength of many other species. Just as a house cat will never become as large or as strong as an African lion no matter what it eats. But if it eats the best possible diet, and receives all the nutrients it needs, it should grow to be larger and stronger than most other cats of its breed, even without exercise.

I believe my remedies and diet recommendations will work well for everyone, but especially for athletes. The athlete who is relatively free of toxins, and is receiving the nutrients and enzymes that most others are deficient in, would certainly have a tremendous advantage over the competition.

AGING

Another possible benefit from eliminating toxins and ensuring adequate supplies of nutrients is slower aging. It makes sense to me that many people look and feel old too soon in life due in part to toxins. The combination of a poor diet plus toxins in the body equals a recipe for premature aging.

This vicious cycle, if continued, only gets worse as the years go by. New toxins are always continuing to enter our bodies. Our bodies then become overloaded to the point that we can no longer handle the resulting maladies. So, in the Western world, we go to the doctor for prescriptions, which only mask the symptoms. Pharmaceutical medications only give us temporary relief at best, but this adds even more toxins increasing the stress overload on the body.

Studies have found that when a sugar molecule combines with a protein molecule in the body, it disrupts the lower layer of the skin and causes inflammation. This is a process called Glycation. The collagen fibers become cross-linked and that is what actually causes wrinkles to form. The amino acids Arginine and Lysine in the diet bind with the sugar, making it unavailable to act with the collagen protein. This minimizes the inflammation and cross-linking, and results in the formation of fewer wrinkles.

Naturally occurring enzymes in the skin, called MMPs (Matrix Metalloproteinase enzymes), are continually breaking down collagen, elastin, and hyaluronic acid. Collagen gives our skin its strength. Elastin is responsible for the elasticity of the skin, and hyaluronic acid keeps our skin hydrated. Some of the phenolics that are important cofactors in herbs are also great MMPs inhibitors. As we age, our body's resistance to these enzymes decreases and the process increases more rapidly. By the time we reach age 30, we begin to lose 1% of our collagen every year. So by age 50 we have lost approximately 20%, by age 60, approximately 30% and so on.[30]

In my opinion, the rate at which this occurs can be drastically reduced by ridding the body of unwanted toxins and ensuring adequate supplies of nutrients, such as vitamins, minerals, amino acids, phytonutrients, and both digestive and metabolic enzymes. Just because this aging process is what happens to most people does not mean it is inevitable.

BIBLICAL PERSPECTIVE

Our bodies require many nutrients each day to maintain optimum health. In order for this to happen, we need to maintain necessary levels of vitamin C, B vitamins, calcium, magnesium, and many others. My focus has been mainly on identifying the nutrients necessary for detoxification. I have discovered a total of thirty-six various nutrients needed for continual detoxification on a daily basis. They consist of vitamins, minerals, trace elements, amino acids, phenolics, digestive and metabolic enzymes. All of these nutrients will be covered in the following chapters. In my opinion, the most important nutrients in this list are the digestive enzymes.

A high level of digestive enzymes allows for the proper assimilation of all the other nutrients. They are vitally important to proper health. Just like a recipe needs all the ingredients in precise amounts, if one enzyme is missing, or at too low a level, then the entire nutrient combination is thrown out of balance. This will result in a body system which is ineffective at detoxification and ineffective at maintaining good health.

I would like to share my thoughts about why man must deal with toxins. The book of Genesis describes man's longevity after the fall of Adam and Eve in the

Garden of Eden. Man typically lived to be hundreds of years old. Perhaps the Earth was a more hospitable place.

The climate and weather were possibly more ideal, and the Earth could have had a constant temperature day and night. There was probably more oxygen in our atmosphere, thus less of a toxin problem. Disease-causing microbes cannot survive as well with a high level of oxygen. Man was also probably somehow protected from the sun's harmful rays. The food was likely supplied with all the necessary nutrients. All these factors may have contributed to longer life spans.

Genesis 6:3 says, "And the LORD said, My spirit shall not always strive with man, for that he also is flesh: yet his days shall be an hundred and twenty years." After the Great Flood, man's lifespan shortened from 950 years to 175 years in 10 generations. This was from Noah to Abraham. Genesis 9:29 says that Noah lived to be 950 years old. Genesis 11:10–11 says his son Shem lived to be 600 years old.

Shem begat Arphaxad, who lived to be 438 years old. Arphaxad begat Salah, who lived to be 433. Salah begat Eber, who lived to be 464. Eber begat Peleg, who then lived to be 239. Peleg begat Re'u, who lived to be 239. Re'u begat Serug, who lived to be 230. Serug begat Nahor, who lived to be 148. Nahor begat Terah, who lived to be 205. Terah begat Abram, who lived to be 175.

Through my testing, I have found that there are just a few digestive enzymes that are not plentiful in our food supply, yet are necessary for detoxification. They are not completely missing - they are just not plentiful. Most of the foods which do contain them supply them in low levels. These low levels are not enough to give one the maximum benefit for utilizing other nutrients. In my opinion, we need high levels of all digestive enzymes on a daily basis. The metabolic enzymes can be at low levels, and they are typically found that way. My theory is that after the Great Flood, perhaps enzymes were no longer plentiful in our food supply. Added to this was the fact that the Earth was no longer an ideal place to live. Man had to deal with exposure to the sun's harmful rays, an unsteady climate, temperature extremes, and harmful microbes. This, is of course, only my speculation.

I am basing my ideas on the biblical account of that time in history, plus what I have found through my testing. In Genesis 3:22, God mentions the Tree of Life where man could eat of it and live forever. That was one of the reasons he sent Adam and Eve from the Garden. As punishment for man's sin, God did not want man to live forever. I hypothesize the Tree of Life bore fruit which contained all of the nutrients man would need for optimum health.

This fruit no longer exists, but I believe we are able to receive adequate amounts of all the nutrients we need through careful diet and proper supplementation. My testing has convinced me that we can receive all of our enzymes and cofactors through eating meat, dairy, eggs, nuts, seeds, and fruits. It does not take much imagination for me to see that God could have easily created a fruit which contained all of the necessary digestive and metabolic enzymes, plus all of the necessary cofactors.

This fruit would have protected man from toxins by containing all of the adequate amounts of enzymes and cofactors. Man would not need to worry about disease from bacteria, fungi, viruses, or parasites. I do not believe humans would even be adversely affected from a venomous bite. Animals probably did not eat flesh at this point, either. They would have basically eaten what man did, so they would have also been protected from the same harmful microbes. I have tested enough animal blood samples to know that they also have to deal with the same toxin problems as man.

I would like to give my version of what I believe the world was like before and after the Flood. After Adam and Eve where removed from the Garden, they had to work for their food, meaning they had to tend their crops and animals. I do not believe man ate meat at this point. I do believe man was created to be an omnivore from the very beginning, but most of his food was probably fruit from trees. I do believe man may have included eggs and milk in his diet, but not flesh.

In Genesis 1: 29–30 God says, "Behold, I have given you every herb bearing seed, which *is* upon the face of all the earth, and every tree, in the which *is* the fruit of a tree yielding seed; to you it shall be for meat.[30] And to every beast of the earth, and to every fowl of the air, and to every thing that creepeth upon the earth, wherein *there is* life, *I have given* every green herb for meat: and it was so."

The Bible says in Genesis 2:15–17 And the Lord God took the man, and put him into the garden of Eden to dress it and to keep it."[16] "And the LORD God commanded the man, saying, Of every tree of the garden thou mayest freely eat:[17] but of the tree of the knowledge of good and evil, thou shalt not eat of it: for in the day that thou eatest thereof thou shalt surely die."

After Adam and Eve sinned, Genesis 3:17–19 says, "cursed *is* the ground for thy sake; in sorrow shalt thou eat of it all the days of thy life;[18] thorns also and thistles shall it bring forth to thee; and thou shalt eat the herb of the field:[19] in the sweat of thy face shalt thou eat bread,"

Then in Genesis 3:22–24 the Bible mentions the Tree of Life: "And the Lord God said, Behold, the man is become as one of us, to know good and evil: and now, lest he put forth his hand, and take also of the tree of life, and eat, and live for ever:[23] therefore the Lord God sent him forth from the garden of Eden, to till the ground from whence he was taken.[24] So he drove out the man: and he placed at the east of the garden of Eden cherubim, and a flaming sword which turned every way, to keep the way of the tree of life.

I believe at this point that even though man had to work for his food, meaning planting and tending crops, I think it was probably easy to grow food.

Genesis 2:5–6 says, "…for the Lord God had not caused it to rain upon the earth, and *there was* not a man to till the ground.[6] But there went up a mist from the earth, and watered the whole face of the ground."

I would imagine the Earth of Adam's day could be described as being more of a tropical setting, similar to the climate around the equator today. I suspect it had a very pleasant temperature and was very green with much vegetation. I would also imagine it was very easy to grow all types of food since man did not have to worry about watering his crops.

Based upon the Scriptures, I do not think there was much rock visible. Everything would have probably been covered with soil and grass. All of this is a bit hard to imagine today since the part of the world where the Garden of Eden was located is mostly very dry and considered more of a desert region. Most mountain peaks are very rocky all the way down to the tree line, which is about 12,000 feet. Man was probably living at a much higher altitude, so there were no mountains like we have today. I would speculate that sea level would have been several thousand feet higher than it is now. There was probably not as much land available. It was mostly under water, so the oceans would have been much deeper than they currently are.

Genesis 7:19–20 says, "And the waters prevailed exceedingly upon the earth; and all the high hills, that *were* under the whole heaven, were covered.[20] Fifteen cubits upward did the waters prevail; and the mountains were covered."

Fifteen cubits is not very deep water. This is why I do not believe man lived at the lower elevations like he does today. Genesis 8:4 states that Noah's ark landed in the mountains of Ararat which reach elevations of above 16,000 feet.

Genesis 9:2–3 says, "And the fear of you and the dread of you shall be upon every beast of the earth, and upon every fowl of the air, upon all that moveth *upon* the earth, and upon all the fishes of the sea; into your hand are they delivered.[3] Every moving thing that liveth shall be meat for you; even as the green herb have I given you all things.

This is the point at which I believe both man and animal started to eat flesh. God essentially gave permission. Noah and his family would have continued to basically eat the same diet that they were used to eating before the flood, but food was no longer plentiful. It would be much more difficult to grow crops and much easier to kill and eat animals for food. But there is no indication God ever changed man or animals, only their environment.

Part of Genesis 6:3 says, "And the Lord said, My spirit shall not always strive with man." I believe what God meant by, "strive with man," was that spiritually He would remove some of his protection from man. Before the flood, man was free to roam the earth without fear of being attacked by animals we now consider predators.

I like to use the analogy of the fact that our atmosphere is naturally cold. The only warmth the Earth receives is from the sun. When it is warm outside it is not from a lack of cold. It is still there, it is just being pushed aside temporarily by the sun's heat; as soon as the sun is gone, it becomes cold again. The same is true in a spiritual sense - the only good we receive comes from God. When God is gone, evil takes over.

Before the Great Flood, there was probably no such thing as hunger. Food was everywhere and plentiful. Neither man nor animals needed to view each other as possible meals. I suspect man continued to eat more of a vegetarian diet for generations after the flood. This would have been the dietary habit passed on from Noah's family, but since fruit was possibly no longer plentiful, man would not always be in an environment where he could have it readily available to him.

Weather conditions were no longer always ideal for growing fruit. Of course, the colder climates would not allow people to grow many crops at all. As man spread out to inhabit more areas of the Earth, he would turn to whatever source of food that was most easily available to him. The warmer climates had more ideal conditions for growing a variety of crops, but the knowledge of what man needed to eat for optimum health was no longer available. Man became mainly interested in survival, not health. After a few generations had passed, I do not believe anyone remembered the diet of Noah's generation. I also feel certain that Noah's generation did not understand how much their diet protected them. It was not until the late 1800's that man even became aware of germs and the effect they have on our bodies.

Man's dietary needs have never changed. He still needs the same diet for proper health that Adam and Eve had. The question has always been, "What exactly is that diet?" Our food is probably somewhat different now from what it was then. I believe our food today has a lower level of nutrition than the food before the Flood. However, I believe we can achieve great health results if we consume the foods containing the highest levels of nutrients. I will cover what nutrients I have found man needs in the following chapters.

FINAL THOUGHTS ON REMEDIES

Many alternative health companies are, of course, interested in finding alternative treatments and possible cures for diseases that do not involve using traditional medicine because of potential harmful side effects. As a result, many times they are looking "out there" somewhere to find answers. The "out there" could be under the ocean, at the North and South poles, or even the Amazon jungle. I believe that we have everything we need right here in front of us and we just don't realize it yet.

Various companies are continually doing research to find new and different nutrients and antioxidants, which is a good thing. The more we can learn and understand about nutrition, the healthier we will all be. However, the problem is that every new nutrient and antioxidant found suddenly becomes "the new fad" for the next few months, or even years. Health companies start packaging and promoting them to health food stores so they will in turn buy and then sell them to the general public. Many of these nutrients may not be assimilated properly by our bodies without the right enzymes. Our bodies need to take in the right amount of the proper enzymes for peak performance. My opinion is that we have the technology to find all of this information, but we are not using this newly revealed information to our best advantage.

A good starting point is to determine what nutrients are needed, and in what amounts for detoxification and optimum health. The USDA (United States Department of Agriculture) has already started this process by establishing the RDA (Recommended Dietary Allowance) with many, but not all, nutrients. The RDA has been determined for vitamins, minerals, and amino acids, but not digestive and metabolic enzymes or phytonutrients. Once these can be determined and established we can then focus on the best possible sources for each.

This is what I have done in my testing. In the following section of this book I will list thirty-six nutrients I have found which I believe are necessary for optimum health. Eighteen of them are enzymes and the remaining eighteen are their cofactors. They are each listed by category in alphabetical order. I will also list what herbs and foods contain each of them and which ones contain them at the highest levels.

NUTRIENTS

nu·tri·ent (nü-trē-ənt) **n.** [L. *nutrire* "nourish"]. Any substance that can be metabolized by an organism to give energy and build tissue. Any element or compound that is necessary for or contributes to an organism's metabolism, growth, or other functioning. **adj.** nourishing; providing nourishment or nutriment.

Random House Dictionary, Random House, Inc., 2006

The American Heritage Science Dictionary, Houghton Mifflin Company, 2002.

ENZYMES

Enzymes are proteins that accelerate, or catalyze, the chemical reactions of living cells. This happens in both plants and animals. Catalysis is the increased rate of a chemical reaction induced by a substance called a catalyst. As with all catalysts, enzymes are not consumed by the reactions they catalyze. Without enzymes, most biochemical reactions would be too slow to carry on the process of life.

Throughout history, people have made use of enzyme-catalyzed reactions. For example, the processes for brewing, baking, and producing medications are all enzyme-catalyzed reactions. Many drugs work by activating or inhibiting a particular enzyme. Isolated enzymes are also commonly used in the textile, leather, food, and beverage industries. Artificial enzymes, called enzyme mimics, are also designed and produced for industrial and research purposes.

The manufacture of enzymes is regulated by the cell's genetic material, deoxyribonucleic acid (DNA), through the process of protein synthesis. Protein synthesis is the creation of proteins using DNA and RNA (ribonucleic acid). The ability of a cell to grow and divide is mainly determined by the number and different kinds of enzymes it contains. Several hundred different reactions may happen simultaneously within a cell, and each is catalyzed by one or more enzymes. All cells contain enzymes capable of catalyzing the synthesis of thousands of protein molecules in a second. There are over one thousand different enzymes found in a human cell. Digestive enzymes break down the carbohydrates, proteins and fats in our diet and allow us to benefit from the nutrients in our food.

While this is happening, enzymes are also removing toxins, which are then eliminated as waste. Metabolic enzymes speed up the chemical reaction within the cells for detoxification and energy production. They enable us to see, hear, feel, move, and think. Our bodies naturally produce both digestive and metabolic enzymes as they are needed.[31] Surplus enzymes are stored by some organs for later use and used as fuel for the brain. In order for an enzyme to perform all of its necessary functions, it needs cofactors. Enzymes are catalysts for cells and cofactors are catalysts for enzymes. Removal of the cofactor from the enzyme's structure causes the loss of its catalytic activity.

Some enzymes are able to function without the need of any additional components, or cofactors. I have found through my testing that some of the metabolic enzymes will digest many toxins without needing cofactors. Sometimes combining several enzymes together works similar to having cofactors. However, in order to function to their full ability, most enzymes need cofactors.

An enzyme without a cofactor is referred to as an apoenzyme. An apoenzyme is the protein component of an enzyme which requires a cofactor for activity. Once the cofactor attaches, the enzyme becomes active and is then referred to as a holoenzyme. Cofactors can be divided into two groups: coenzymes and prosthetic groups. Basically, the difference between the two groups is that coenzymes are not permanently bound to the enzyme while the prosthetic group is permanently bound to the enzyme.[32]

I am convinced that if a person has a health issue, they are most likely experiencing two problems. They probably have a toxin, or multiple toxins, and they are also deficient in one or more enzymes. In my opinion, the toxins are really secondary to the nutritional deficiency. Lacking the right nutrition, as well as the correct quantity of that nutrition, is the primary health issue. If a person has the right nutrition and the correct amount of it, they will not have many toxins in their body. Toxins will not be able to stay in their body, because they will be digested by the enzymes and cofactors. Any toxins that are alive, such as a parasite, will not be able to live in a body with the right nutrition. Any toxins that are not living organisms, such as chemicals, will be flushed out or digested by the proper nutrition.

The following pages will cover digestive and metabolic enzymes. I will describe each enzyme, its function, and some of the herbs and foods in which it can be found. I will then do the same with each individual cofactor. I would also like to add that the foods listed do contain other nutrients. I have chosen to list only the thirty-six nutrients in these foods which have shown from my testing to be necessary for detoxification. This does not mean the other nutrients are less important. It also does not mean the other nutrients do not play a part in the detoxification process. Their role is probably more of an indirect one. I am only concerned with the detoxification capabilities of these foods for the purpose of this book.

Digestive Enzymes

Digestion is defined as the ability to convert food into a form that can be properly assimilated by the body. Digestive enzymes are secreted along the digestive tract to break down food into nutrients and waste. This allows the nutrients to be absorbed, or assimilated, into the blood stream and the waste to be discarded. Nutrients can only be delivered to the cells by enzymes.

Many people consume specialty supplements, not realizing that enzymes are needed to deliver the nutrients. Thus, the supplements are taken in vain, wasted, because the nutrients could not be used by the cells because the delivery mechanism was not present. When the person taking the supplement does not get the expected benefits, the person assumes that an even larger amount is needed by the body for the desired results. The truth is that in most cases the body only needs small amounts of nutrients with high levels of digestive enzymes.[33] It is impossible to consume enough supplements to satisfy our body's nutrient requirements without digestive enzymes. Think of your mail - you get your mail because it is delivered by the mailman. The same is true of nutrients - the enzymes "deliver" the nutrients to your cells.

Through my testing I have found fourteen primary digestive enzymes necessary for detoxification. I will describe each of them and list some of the herbs and foods that contain them.

Amylase

Amylase enzymes are present in all types of organs and tissues. They are also found in parts of plants. In animals, the highest concentrations are found in saliva and the pancreas. The main function of Amylase is to be a catalyst in the breakdown, or hydrolysis, of starch into simple sugars such as maltose. During the ripening of fruit, amylase breaks starch into sugar, resulting in the sweet flavor of ripe fruit.[34]

My testing shows that amylase helps in the assimilation of phytonutrients.

HERBS	FOODS
Fennel	Peanuts
Ginger	Raspberries
	Strawberries
	Sunflower Seeds
	Walnuts

Bromelain

Bromelain is an enzyme found in the pineapple and related plants of the family Bromelidaceae, which hydrolyze proteins. They are available as byproducts from commercial pineapple production, usually from the stems, and are used to tenderize meat, and to treat sausage casings.

Similar enzymes are found in figs and pawpaw plants, such as ficain and papain. Bromelain has been proposed in the use of arthritis, gout, hemorrhoids, and ulcerative colitis. Studies have shown that it can be useful in the reduction of platelet clumping and blood clots in the bloodstream.[35]

My testing shows bromelain to help in the assimilation of phytonutrients.

HERBS	FOODS
N/A	Cacao
	Pineapple
	Raspberries
	Salmonberries
	Strawberries
	Walnuts

Cellulase

Cellulase refers to a group of enzymes which, acting together, work as catalysts in the breakdown of cellulose to beta-glucose (blood sugar).[36] Cellulase enzymes are present in intestinal bacteria, and are necessary for the digestion of fiber.

From my testing, I have found that cellulase is an enzyme which helps us to assimilate the phytonutrients and amino acids from our food.

HERBS	FOODS
Fennel	Cacao
Ginger	Eggs
	Peanuts
	Raspberries
	Shrimp
	Strawberries

Intrinsic Factor

Intrinsic factor is necessary for the absorption of vitamin B12. Upon entering the stomach, vitamin B12 binds to one of two binding proteins found in the gastric juice. In the small intestine, other enzymes digest these proteins from the vitamin and allow it to bind to intrinsic factor.

An insufficient supply of this enzyme will not allow benefit from vitamin B12 intake because the vitamin will not absorb through the wall of the small intestine. This can lead to a condition called pernicious anemia.[37]

My testing has revealed intrinsic factor to be in a wide variety of foods. My testing has also shown that intrinsic factor is important to the assimilation of vitamins, minerals, and phytonutrients.

HERBS	FOODS
Corn Silk	Almonds
Ginger	Figs
Witch Hazel	Peanuts
Yerba Santa	Pomegranates
Yucca	Raspberries
	Safflower Oil
	Salmonberries
	Sesame Seeds
	Strawberries
	Watermelons

Lipase

Lipase enzymes are water-soluble enzymes that catalyze the hydrolysis of fats into glycerol and fatty acids. They are present in the pancreatic juice, liver, and adipose tissue. They are found in many seeds and grains. Lipase enzymes are capable of degrading lipid molecules and are sometimes responsible for the development of rancidity in stored foods.[38] People who have constant food cravings, problems with blood sugar, and problems controlling their weight, are probably lacking in lipase enzymes.

My testing has shown lipase to be important to the assimilation of phytonutrients.

HERBS	FOODS
N/A	Cacao
	Raspberries
	Strawberries
	Sunflower Seeds
	Walnuts

Maltase

Maltase is an enzyme produced by the surface cells lining the small intestine. Specifically, it is a catalyst in the breakdown of disaccharide maltose to glucose.[39]

My testing has shown maltase to be the most prevalent digestive enzyme, and it is in a wide variety of foods. Maltase tests as being important to the assimilation of vitamins, minerals, amino acids, and phenolics.

HERBS	FOODS
Fennel	Albacore
Ginger	Cayenne Pepper
	Chicken
	Cinnamon
	Eggs
	Peanuts
	Pineapple
	Raspberries
	Strawberries
	Turkey
	Watermelons
	Zucchini

Pancreatin

Pancreatin is a mixture of several digestive enzymes produced by the exocrine cells of the pancreas. Exocrine glands are glands that secrete enzymes into ducts. They are counterparts to endocrine glands which secrete hormones directly into the bloodstream. It is composed of amylase, lipase, protease, and trypsin. Pancreatin is sometimes referred to as pancreatic acid.[40]

My testing shows pancreatin to be beneficial to the assimilation of both minerals and phytonutrients.

HERBS	**FOODS**
N/A	Raspberries
	Strawberries
	Sunflower Seeds
	Walnuts

Papain

Papain is a proteolytic digestive enzyme usually found in the papaya plant. Proteolytic comes from the word proteolysis, which is the hydrolytic breakdown of proteins into simpler, more soluble substances. Papain catalyzes the lysis of proteins. Lysis refers to the death of a cell by the breaking of its cellular membrane. Papain is used as a meat tenderizer, and in medicine as a digestive aid.[41]

Papain tests as aiding in the assimilation of vitamins and minerals.

HERBS	FOODS
N/A	Cacao
	Papaya
	Pineapple
	Strawberries
	Walnuts

Pepsin

Pepsin is a proteolytic digestive enzyme released by the gastric chief cells, or peptic cells, in the stomach. Its purpose is to catalyze the breakdown of food proteins into peptides. The link between one amino acid and the next is known as an amide bond, or a peptic bond. Proteins are polypeptide molecules, meaning they consist of many subunits bound together by peptides. Pepsin is prepared commercially for food manufacturing, and as a digestive aid.[42]

My testing has shown pepsin to aid in the assimilation of minerals.

HERBS	FOODS
N/A	Cacao
	Cinnamon
	Strawberries
	Walnuts

Potassium Bicarbonate

Potassium bicarbonate (KHC03) is a colorless, odorless, salty-tasting substance that is soluble in water. It occurs as a soft white granular powder or in crystal form. Potassium bicarbonate is found throughout nature in living and non-living environments. It is an integral part of the normal function of animals, plants and virtually all living organisms.[43]

It is best known for its use in baking powder and as an antacid. Commercially, it is also used as a fire retardant in powder fire extinguishers for crops to neutralize the acidity of the soil, and it is added to bottled water for taste.

My testing has shown potassium bicarbonate to be useful in the assimilation of minerals.

HERBS	FOODS
N/A	Baking Powder
	Cayenne Pepper
	Cinnamon
	Raspberries
	Walnuts

Protease

Protease is any enzyme that performs proteolysis, or protein digestion. It starts protein catabolism by hydrolysis of the peptide bonds that link amino acids together in the polypeptide chain. Catabolism is the chemical reaction which breaks down molecules into smaller units and releases energy. Proteases occur naturally in all organisms and our immune systems are in constant need of them. Toxins, such as bacteria, excrete proteins, or exotoxins, which can damage cells and disrupt normal cellular metabolism.[44] There are currently six classifications of protease enzymes.

My testing shows protease to aid in the assimilation of phytonutrients.

HERBS	FOODS
N/A	Cacao
	Cayenne Pepper
	Raspberries
	Strawberries
	Sunflower Seeds
	Walnuts

Ribonuclease

Ribonuclease, (RNase), is a group of enzymes ubiquitous in living organisms and is exceptionally stable. They can be divided into endoribonucleases and exoribonucleases. Their main function is to catalyze the hydrolysis of ribonucleic acid (RNA) into smaller components. This happens by the enzymes removing the nucleotides from either end of the RNA molecule.[45]

Through my testing, I have found ribonuclease to assist with the assimilation of vitamins, minerals and amino acids.

HERBS	FOODS
N/A	Beef
	Cacao
	Eggs
	Lamb
	Milk
	Pork
	Raspberries
	Strawberries
	Walnuts

Sodium Bicarbonate

Sodium bicarbonate (NaHC03) is a white solid that is crystalline, but appears as a fine powder. It is a water-soluble component of the mineral natron. The natural mineral form is called nahcolite. Natron is a naturally-occurring compound mixture of sodium carbonate and sodium bicarbonate. Like potassium bicarbonate, sodium bicarbonate is also found throughout nature.[46]

Both potassium bicarbonate and sodium bicarbonate are crucial to the normal functions of both animals and plants. The commercial uses of sodium bicarbonate are primarily for cooking and baking, as in baking soda. It is also used in medicine as an antacid. Both are also produced artificially for many uses.

My testing reveals that sodium bicarbonate helps with the assimilation of minerals.

<u>HERBS</u>	<u>FOODS</u>
N/A	Baking Soda
	Brewer's Yeast
	Cayenne Pepper
	Strawberries
	Walnuts

Trypsin

Trypsin is a protease enzyme that falls under the classification of serine proteases. It is produced in the pancreas, and then secreted into the duodenum. Trypsin works to catalyze the hydrolysis of proteins into smaller peptides or amino acids.[47] Trypsin is used in medicine to treat blood clots, and also commercially in baby food to pre-digest it.

My testing shows that trypsin helps with the assimilation of minerals and phytonutrients.

HERBS	FOODS
N/A	Cacao
	Pineapple
	Raspberries
	Strawberries
	Sunflower Seeds
	Walnuts

Metabolic Enzymes

Enzymes enable all of the many chemical reactions to take place at any second inside of a plant or an animal. There are three basic types of enzymes: food enzymes, digestive enzymes, and metabolic enzymes. Our diet contains food enzymes which aid in the process of digestion. They set in motion the digestive process as soon as food enters the mouth. As these enzymes move with the food into the upper portion of the stomach, they continue to assist with digestion.

Our bodies produce digestive enzymes which facilitate the conversion of food to energy, as well as aid in a variety of other necessary biological functions. The digestive glands secrete juices containing enzymes that break down nutrients chemically into smaller molecules that are more easily absorbed by the body. Our bodies also produce metabolic enzymes, which are the largest of all enzyme types. We can also obtain metabolic enzymes from our diet. They assist in a wide range of basic bodily processes, from breathing to thinking. Some metabolic enzymes are devoted to maintaining the immune system by repairing damaged cells. Others are involved in controlling the harmful effects of toxins by converting them into forms that the body can expel more easily.

Every organ, tissue, and cell in our body relies on the reaction of metabolic enzymes. They are produced in the liver, gallbladder, pancreas, and other organs.[48] My testing has proven to me the importance of metabolic enzymes by demonstrating that they digest the toxins we are continually encountering. On the following pages I will be covering four primary metabolic enzymes necessary for detoxification and some of the herbs and foods in which they are found.

Phosphomannose Isomerase

Phosphommanose Isomerase (PMI) is a metabolic enzyme that is not very common in plants. It is sometimes referred to as mannose phosphate isomerase. It functions to catalyze the conversion of mannose-6-phosphate (M6P) to fructose-6-phosphate. Mannose is converted to mannose-6-phosphate and then PMI converts it to fructose-6-phosphate. Most fructose and glucose are converted to fructose 6-phosphate.[49]

A lack of this enzyme in humans results in a disease called Carbohydrate-Deficient Glycoprotein Syndrome (CDGS). CDGS is an inherited metabolic disorder that may be mistaken for Cerebral Palsy. The major symptoms include intolerance for fructose (Fructosemia), galactose (Galactosemia), and low blood sugar (Hypoglycemia).[50]

My testing has shown this enzyme to be rare, but so very important to detoxification. It tests as being helpful in detoxifying radiation.

HERBS	FOODS
Fennel	Peanuts
Ginger	Raspberries
Sheep Sorrel	Strawberries

Superoxide Dismutase

Superoxide dismutase (SOD) is a metabolic enzyme that catalyzes the dismutation of superoxide into oxygen and hydrogen peroxide. Dismutation is a chemical reaction in which an element is simultaneously reduced and oxidized to form two different products. Oxidation is the loss of electrons, and reduction is the gain of electrons. To state it more simply, SOD inactivates superoxide free-radicals and prevents them from damaging cell membranes.[51] This is why SOD is an important antioxidant defense in nearly all cells exposed to oxygen.

My testing has revealed that SOD is not very abundant in common herbs and foods. It tests as helping to eliminate bacteria, parasites, and heavy metals. SOD does appear to occur naturally in fungi.

HERBS	FOODS
Elecampane	Garlic
Slippery Elm	Soybeans
Uva Ursi	Strawberries
Yucca	

Urokinase

Urokinase (Abbokinase) is a metabolic enzyme that catalyzes the conversion of plasminogen to plasmin and is used in medicine to dissolve blood clots. It is sometimes referred to as urokinase-type Plasminogen Activator (uPA). Plasminogen is the inactive precursor to plasmin that is found in body fluids and blood plasma.

Plasmin is an important enzyme present in the blood that degrades many blood plasma proteins. The most common proteins that plasmin dissolve are fibrin clots. The degradation of fibrin is called fibrinolysis.[52] I frequently find urokinase in many herbs and foods.

My testing has revealed its importance in helping to detoxify viruses and vaccine residue. My testing has also revealed that urokinase occurs naturally in both bacteria and fungi.

HERBS	FOODS
Corn Silk	Canola Oil
Echinacea Ang.	Cayenne Pepper
Plantain	Cinnamon
Witch Hazel	Oregano
Yerba Santa	Raspberries
	Sesame Seeds
	Sunflower Seeds

Baker's Yeast Enzyme (Saccharomyces cerevisiae)

Baker's yeast is the common name for the strain of yeast Saccharomyces cerevisiae.[53] It is commonly used as a leavening agent in baking. My testing has demonstrated that the enzymes found in baker's yeast are the most common metabolic enzymes found in herbs.[54]

Out of all the many herbs I have tested, baker's yeast enzyme was revealed as a component almost 50% of the time. It also tests as being the most critical enzyme for detoxifying all the various organic and inorganic toxins. It tests as helping to detoxify fungi, venoms, and chemicals.

HERBS	FOODS
Aloe	Cacao
Artemisia	Olives
Black Walnut	Sesame Seeds
Comfrey	Strawberries
Goldenseal	
Grapefruit Seed Extract	
Plantain	
Senna	
Valerian	
Witch Hazel	

VITAMINS

Vitamins are organic compounds required in only tiny amounts for essential metabolic reactions. Most vitamins cannot be obtained in sufficient quantities by synthesis in the body, so they must also be acquired through the diet. Vitamin deficiencies can cause specific diseases. For example, a vitamin D deficiency can cause a condition known as rickets. Vitamin D is important to the absorption of calcium and phosphorous. This makes it essential for having strong, healthy bones and teeth.[55]

Vitamins are usually considered coenzymes, which are classified as a type of cofactor, because their action is to transport chemical groups from one enzyme to another. Cofactors are non-protein chemical compounds that are tightly bound to an enzyme and are required for catalysis. In a broader sense, coenzymes are considered a type of cofactor. When cofactors are bound to an enzyme they are called prosthetic groups.

Coenzymes are non-protein molecules that do not form a permanent part of the enzyme's structure like a prosthetic group does. Coenzymes are released from the enzyme's active site during the catalytic reaction. Vitamins can serve as precursors to coenzymes, or as the coenzymes themselves. For example, niacin is a precursor to the coenzyme nicotinamide adenine dinucleotide (NAD). Vitamin C, on the other hand, acts as a coenzyme itself. Cofactors can be either inorganic, e.g. metal ions, or organic, e.g. vitamins and minerals.[56]

My testing has demonstrated that vitamins are not as directly important to detoxification as one might think. Out of the thirty-six nutrients I have found necessary for detoxifying, only one vitamin has shown up consistently– Vitamin B8. While vitamins are important for support in growth, healing, and maintaining good health, they appear to be less important for detoxification. The role of vitamins in detoxification is more of an indirect one. On the following page I will describe vitamin B8 in detail, and list some of the herbs and foods which contain it.

Inositol

Technically, inositol is not really considered a vitamin because it can be synthesized by the body. The most prominent naturally-occurring form of inositol is myo-inositol. Myo-inositol is considered part of the vitamin B complex and is referred to as vitamin B8. Vitamin B8 is synthesized by the human body from glucose-6-phosphate (G-6-P). Myo-inositol has been found in studies to be effective in treating ailments such as obsessive-compulsive disorder (OCD), and bipolar depression.[57]

My testing has shown inositol to be helpful in the detoxification of heavy metals and vaccine residue.

HERBS	FOODS
Fennel	Beef
Ginger	Peanuts
	Salmonberries

MINERALS

The primary requirements for survival of living organisms are the elements carbon, hydrogen, nitrogen, and oxygen, as well as minerals. The term minerals can refer to the inorganic heavy metal form of minerals, or the organic ions found in food. An inorganic mineral is a naturally occurring solid with a definite chemical composition and a specific crystalline structure. Rocks are typically a combination of inorganic minerals.

Organic minerals are present in virtually every cell of the body. They help maintain general homeostasis and are required for normal functioning. Acute imbalances of minerals can be potentially fatal. Minerals contribute to good health as long as they are from an organic source. Plants absorb minerals from the soil and process them to become ionic so that our body can assimilate them easily. Minerals from an inorganic source, such as heavy metals, cannot be used by the body and thus accumulate in the tissues.

Organic minerals are classified as either macrominerals or microminerals. Obviously, macrominerals are required in relatively large amounts, and microminerals, or trace minerals, are required in relatively minute amounts. Examples of macrominerals are calcium, magnesium, potassium, sodium and phosphorous. Examples of microminerals are manganese, selenium, vanadium, silicon, and chromium. Many trace minerals play an important role in the catalysis of enzymes. For example, selenium is required for the catalysis of peroxidase enzymes.

Some macrominerals are referred to as electrolytes. Electrolytes are free ions that behave as electrically conductive mediums. They commonly exist as solutions, such as salt in water. When an organic mineral, such as sodium chloride, comes into contact with water, it breaks down into sodium ions and chloride ions. Ions are atoms or molecules that have lost or gained one or more electrons. This would give it either a positive or a negative charge. This reaction is referred to as solvation, or dissolution, which means the salt is dissolving in the water and creating a solution that conducts electricity.[58]

My testing has shown repeatedly the importance of minerals as cofactors to enzymes. In the following pages I will cover three primary macrominerals and four primary trace minerals that I have found to be important to detoxification. I will describe each of them and list some of the herbs and foods which contain them.

Potassium Chloride

Potassium chloride (KCI) is a chemical compound composed of potassium and chlorine. It has an odorless crystal structure and is commonly referred to as muriate of potash. Potash is an impure form of potassium carbonate. KCI is used in medicine and food processing.

Potassium chloride is also one of the main components of gastric acid in the stomach. Gastric acid is one of the main secretions in the stomach and consists mainly of hydrochloric acid (HCI), and smaller quantities of potassium chloride (KCI) and sodium chloride (NaCI).[59]

My research has shown KCI to be an abundant mineral found in many herbs and foods. My research has also revealed its importance in helping to eliminate toxins such as bacteria, parasites, venoms, chemicals, heavy metals, and radiation.

HERBS	FOODS
Corn silk	Beef
Comfrey	Cayenne Pepper
Goldenseal	Cinnamon
Plantain	Eggs
Senna	Garlic
Wormwood	Sunflower Seeds
	Walnuts

Sodium Chloride

Sodium chloride (NaCI) is a chemical compound composed of sodium and chlorine. It is most commonly known as table salt. NaCI is the salt most responsible for the salinity of the ocean. NaCI comprises nearly 80% of seawater. Most salt for table use is obtained from seawater. It has many commercial uses from softening water and preserving food to road de-icing. Like potassium chloride, it is also a component of gastric acid in the stomach.[60]

My research has shown sodium chloride to be an abundant mineral found in many herbs and foods. My research has also revealed its contribution in helping to detoxify fungi and vaccine residue.

HERBS	FOODS
Aloe	Beef
Elecampane	Canola Oil
Fennel	Eggs
Ginger	Milk
Valerian Root	Oregano
Witch Hazel	Peanuts
	Sesame Seeds
	Soybeans

Zinc Sulfate

Zinc sulfate (ZnS04) is a water-soluble chemical compound which occurs naturally as the mineral goslarite. It can also be prepared by reacting zinc with aqueous sulfuric acid, or by adding solid zinc to a Copper II Sulfate solution. It is used commercially as a leather preservative, in fertilizers, and in medicine as an astringent and emetic.[61]

This mineral is rare in most common herbs and foods. It tests as helping with the detoxification of viruses and heavy metals.

HERBS	FOODS
Echinacea	Cayenne Pepper
Yerba Santa	Cinnamon
Sheep Sorrel	Eggs
	Walnuts

TRACE ELEMENTS

Technically, a trace element is an element in a sample that has an average concentration of less than 100 parts per million atoms, or less than 100 micrograms per gram. In biochemistry, a trace element is also referred to as a micronutrient, which is a chemical element that is needed in only minute quantities for proper growth and development.

Although only tiny traces of these elements appear to be required for animals, they are much more important to the metabolism of plants. There is still some controversy over how much should be established as a recommended daily intake of certain trace minerals because it is sometimes harder to prove the efficacy of such low concentrations. Fortunately, this is changing due to technological advances. Many trace minerals have been proven to be required components to enzymes as cofactors. The body has the ability to maintain trace minerals within a certain range despite varying intake. This process is called homeostasis. Homeostasis involves the processes of absorption, storage, and excretion.[62]

My testing has shown that it is common for people to be deficient in trace minerals. This is probably due, at least in part, to the presence of toxins. Being deficient in these trace minerals interferes with normal homeostatic regulating functions in the body and causes deficiencies.

On the following pages I will be covering four primary trace minerals I have found to be necessary for detoxification. I will describe each of them and list some of the herbs and foods which contain them.

Selenium

Selenium (Se) is a chemical element necessary in trace amounts for cellular function in most, if not all, animals. Selenium is a necessary cofactor for the antioxidant enzymes glutathione peroxidase and thioredoxin reductase. These enzymes indirectly reduce certain oxidized molecules in animals and some plants. Selenium is also a cofactor for three known deiodinase enzymes, which convert one thyroid hormone to another.[63]

My testing has shown selenium to be an important cofactor in the detoxification of chemicals and parasites.

HERBS	FOODS
Slippery Elm	Cacao
Uva Ursi	Eggs
Yucca	Olives

Silicon

Silicon (Si) is an essential chemical element in biology. Only trace amounts appear to be required by animals, but it is much more important to the metabolism of plants. Various grasses in particular are dependant on silicon for their protective shell. Silicon is the second most abundant element, behind oxygen, making up 25% of the Earth's crust. Silicon is used in making glass, ceramics and cement, and also has many commercial uses in industry as the principal component of most semiconductor devices.[64]

My testing has revealed silicon to be helpful in detoxifying chemicals and heavy metals.

HERBS	FOODS
Elecampane	Cayenne Pepper
Fennel	Cinnamon
Ginger	Milk
Prickly Ash	Peanuts

Titanium

Titanium (Ti) is a chemical element that is considered non-toxic to humans even in large doses. Because inorganic titanium is biocompatible, or non-toxic, it has many uses in medicine. It is used in making surgical implements, joint replacement implants, and dental implants. Titanium appears to be important to the growth of many plants.[65]

My testing shows titanium to be in many common herbs and foods. It also tests as being an important cofactor in detoxifying fungi and radiation.

HERBS	FOODS
Black Walnut	Cacao
Hawthorn	Cinnamon
Sheep Sorrel	Eggs
Witch Hazel	Sesame Seeds
	Soybeans

Vanadium

Vanadium (V) is a chemical element that is one of the twenty-six elements found in most living organisms. Vanadium is an essential component of nitrogenase enzymes. Nitrogenase is the enzyme used by some organisms to catalyze the conversion of atmospheric nitrogen gas to ammonia.

Vanadium deficiencies in animals can result in reduced growth and impaired reproduction. Some forms of vanadium are used to improve glucose control in people with type 2 diabetes. Commercially, vanadium is an important oxidation catalyst.[66]

My testing has shown vanadium to be an abundant trace mineral found in many herbs and foods. My testing has also revealed its importance as a cofactor in helping to eliminate many toxins such as bacteria, viruses, parasites, venoms, and vaccine residue.

HERBS	FOODS
Comfrey	Beef
Corn Silk	Cacao
Echinacea Ang.	Canola Oil
Goldenseal	Cayenne Pepper
Plantain	Garlic
Senna	Sunflower Seeds
Wormwood	Walnuts
Yerba Santa	

AMINO ACIDS

An amino acid is an organic compound made of carbon, hydrogen, oxygen, nitrogen, and in some cases, sulfur, bonded together. Amino acids are considered the building blocks of all living things. They are essential components of our body tissues, organs, nerves, and enzymes. They also help to regulate every biochemical reaction in the body.

All of the millions of different proteins in living things are formed by the bonding of only twenty different amino acids. The human body only produces twelve of these twenty required for manufacturing all of our necessary proteins. This means that we must acquire the remaining eight through our diet. Most plants are able to synthesize all of their amino acids.

Biosynthesis is a vital part of metabolism. Our body synthesizes amino acids from simpler protein compounds by a series of enzymatic reactions. The main chemical reaction that is characteristic of amino acids involves the formation of peptide bonds between two groups of amino acids. Amino acids function as monomers, or individual units, that join together to form large chain-like molecules called polymers.

If there are more than ten amino acids in a chain, it is referred to as a polypeptide. If there are fifty or more, then it is called a protein. The specific properties of each kind of protein are dependant upon the kind and sequence of amino acids. Just as these proteins form when amino acids bond together in long chains, they are also broken down again by hydrolysis in digestion. This is the reverse reaction of the formation of peptide bonds. Digestive enzymes break down the peptide linkage and the amino acids separate again. They are released into the small intestine and pass into the bloodstream and then carried throughout the body. Each individual cell then uses these amino acids to form new and different proteins required for its specific functions.[67]

Through my testing I have found three primary amino acids needed as cofactors to enzymes for detoxification. I will describe each of them and list some of the herbs and foods which contain them.

Threonine

Threonine (Thr) is an essential amino acid, meaning it is not synthesized by the human body and must be supplied by the diet. As a result, we must ingest threonine in the form of threonine-containing proteins. In plants, threonine is synthesized from aspartic acid and homoserine. Aspartic acid and homoserine are amino acids that act as precursors, or intermediates, in the biosynthesis of several amino acids.[68]

In my testing, I have found threonine to be helpful to enzymes in the detoxification of chemicals, parasites, and viruses.

HERBS	FOODS
Corn Silk	Beef
Plantain	Cinnamon
Slippery Elm	Sunflower Seeds
Uva Ursi	Walnuts
Yucca	

Tryptophan

Tryptophan (Trp) is an essential amino acid formed from proteins during digestion by the action of proteolytic enzymes. It is necessary for normal growth and development and is the precursor of serotonin and niacin. Tryptophan is sometimes marketed as 5-Hydroxytryptophan (5-HTP), and is a naturally occurring precursor to serotonin and an intermediate in tryptophan metabolism. It is considered an antidepressant, appetite suppressant, and a sleep aid.[69]

Tryptophan has shown to be an important cofactor mainly in the detoxifying of heavy metals.

HERBS	FOODS
Aloe	Canola Oil
Fennel	Milk
Ginger	Peanuts
Slippery Elm	Turkey

Tyrosine

Tyrosine (Tyr) is a non-essential amino acid used by cells to synthesize proteins. Humans synthesize tyrosine from the essential amino acid phenylalanine. The conversion of phenylalanine to tyrosine is catalyzed by the enzyme phenylalanine hydroxylase. Tyrosine is a precursor of melanin, and the hormones epinephrine, and thyroxine.[70]

I have found tyrosine to be an important cofactor in the detoxification of parasites and radiation.

HERBS	FOODS
Black Walnut	Beef
Corn Silk	Canola Oil
Hawthorne	Sesame Seeds
Plantain	Soybeans
Witch Hazel	Sunflower Seeds
	Walnuts

PHENOLICS

In organic chemistry phenolics, sometimes called phytonutrients or phtochemicals, are a class of chemical compounds found in most plants and animals. When mentioning antioxidants people are usually referring to phenolics. Phenolics are typically considered secondary metabolites because they are not vital to immediate survival, but they are very important to ongoing health.

Primary metabolites, such as vitamins, minerals, and amino acids, are more directly involved with the normal growth, development, and reproduction of an organism. Absence of secondary metabolites does not result in immediate death, but rather in long-term impairment of the organism's ability to survive. One might argue that the typical American diet was designed for survival, not for good health. In my view, the lack of phenolics in our diet is one of the main reasons.

The prefix "phyto" originates from the Greek and means plant, but phytonutrients are found in animal source foods, too. I find it interesting that many times phytonutrients are found at higher levels in animal source foods than in plant source foods. Plants produce phenolics for a variety of reasons. Some are produced for attracting pollinating insects, or some for repelling insect pests.

Other phenolics are produced as protection from disease and environmental stresses.

Phytochemicals have been used by humans for centuries. For example, Hippocrates used white willow leaves to relieve fever. The salicin extracted from white willow bark acts as an anti-inflammatory and pain reliever, and was later synthesized to make aspirin.[71] Out of all the nutrients used as cofactors, I believe phenolics are the most important. They are probably the least understood, and most people do not ingest enough on a daily basis. We need a variety of these nutrients, but also enough quantity of the right ones.

Repeatedly, my research has shown just how important phenolics are to detoxification and our general overall health. Through my testing I have found seven primary phenolics needed as cofactors to enzymes in detoxification. In the following pages I will describe each of them and list some of the herbs and foods which contain them.

Gallic Acid

Gallic acid is an organic acid, also known as 3, 4, 5-trihydroxybenzoic acid. Pure gallic acid is a colorless crystalline organic powder found in tannins. Tannins are astringent, bitter plant polyphenols that are used in tanning animal hides into leather. Gallic acid is used in the pharmaceutical industry to make medicines to treat diabetes, psoriasis, and hemorrhoids.[72]

My testing has shown Gallic acid to be rare in herbs and foods. It does seem to be an important cofactor in helping with the detoxification of vaccine residue.

HERBS	FOODS
Fennel	Cinnamon
Ginger	Eggs
	Peanuts

Urushiol

Urushiol is an oil found in plants of the family Anacardiaceae, such as poison oak and poison ivy. The name comes from the Japanese word urushi. This word comes from the name of a tree grown in East Asia called a kiurushi, which means lacquer tree. A commercial lacquer is produced from this tree.[73]

My testing has shown this phenolic to be very rare in most common herbs and foods, but very important to the detoxification of vaccines.

HERBS	FOODS
Corn Silk	Eggs
	Sunflower Seeds

Valeric Acid

Valeric acid is found naturally in the herb Valerian Root (Valeriana Officinalis), which is also where its name comes from. Sometimes it is referred to as pentanoic acid and has an unpleasant odor. Commercially, it is used for the synthesis of its esters. Esters are a class of chemical compounds used for making perfumes and cosmetics. The process for synthesizing an ester is called esterification, and involves the reaction between an acid and an alcohol.[74]

My testing has shown valeric acid to be rare in most common herbs and foods. It appears to be very important as a cofactor to enzymes in the detoxification of viruses and vaccine residue.

HERBS	FOODS
Corn Silk	Beef
Milk Thistle	Figs
Senna	Oregano
Valerian Root	Strawberries
	Sunflower Seeds

Vanillic Acid

Vanillic acid is an oxidized form of vanillin used as a flavoring agent. Vanillin is the primary component of vanilla extract. Vanillic acid is also a benzoic acid derivative. Benzoic acid is used as a food preservative, and is an important precursor for the synthesis of many other organic substances.[75]

Vanillic acid is a common component of many herbs and foods. My testing has shown it to be an important cofactor for enzymes in detoxifying bacteria, fungi, viruses, parasites, and vaccine residue.

HERBS	FOODS
Echinacea Ang.	Beef
Fennel	Canola Oil
Ginger	Cayenne Pepper
Valerian Root	Cinnamon
Witch Hazel	Peanuts
Yerba Santa	Sesame Seeds
	Vanilla
	Walnuts

Vanillin

Vanillin is an organic compound that is the primary component of the vanilla bean. Synthetic vanillin is used in many foods and pharmaceuticals as a flavoring agent. In addition to vanillin, natural vanilla extract is a mixture of several hundred different compounds. Vanillin is also used to make perfumes, and to mask unpleasant odors of medicines and cleaning products.[76]

Vanillin tests as being a common component of many herbs and foods. It also tests as being an important cofactor to enzymes when detoxifying radiation.

HERBS	FOODS
Fennel	Eggs
Ginger	Peanuts
Uva Ursi	Sesame Seeds
Valerian Root	Vanilla
Witch Hazel	Walnuts
Yucca	

Vanillylamine

Vanillylamine is an organic compound found in many herbs and foods. It is commonly manufactured synthetically and used commercially as a food additive to add pungency to seasonings, flavorings, and spice blends. Vanillylamine is also used in some formulations in the pharmaceutical industry.[77]

My testing has shown it to be an important cofactor for enzymes in detoxifying parasites, viruses, venoms, chemicals, and vaccine residue.

HERBS	FOODS
Corn Silk	Canola Oil
Echinacea Ang.	Cayenne Pepper
Fennel	Cinnamon
Ginger	Eggs
Plantain	Peanuts
Uva Ursi	Sesame Seeds
Valerian Root	Soybeans
Witch Hazel	Sunflower Seeds
Yerba Santa	Vanilla
Yucca	

Xanthine

Xanthine is a natural compound found in most body tissues and plants. Derivatives of xanthine are a group of alkaloids produced by multiple enzyme-catalyzed steps. Alkaloids are chemical derivatives of amino acids.[78] The name alkaloid is derived from the word alkaline. Through my testing I have found xanthine to be a very important component in keeping the body alkaline. Xanthine derivatives are used in the pharmaceutical industry for making mild stimulants, such as bronchodilators and pain relievers.[79]

My testing has shown xanthine to be a component in most herbs and foods. It is an important cofactor for enzymes in eliminating a variety of both organic and inorganic toxins.

HERBS	FOODS
Corn Silk	Beef
Echinacea Ang.	Canola Oil
Fennel	Cayenne Pepper
Ginger	Cinnamon
Plantain	Eggs
Uva Ursi	Milk
Witch Hazel	Olives
Yerba Santa	Peanuts
Yucca	Salmonberries
	Sesame Seeds
	Sunflower Seeds
	Walnuts

NUTRITIONAL RECOMMENDATIONS

In this chapter I summarize my recommended herbs and foods based upon my research. There are many food and herbal combinations a person can consume and still receive all the nutrients necessary for detoxifying and sustaining good health. My recommendation list has the foods and herbs which contain the highest levels of the thirty-six nutrients needed for detoxification and optimum health. A person should be able to eat less food and be more satisfied due to the higher nutritional content.

The digestive enzymes and phenolics are the nutrients which need to be taken at higher levels. I am not suggesting that these are the only foods one should eat, but every diet should include them regularly. For some of the foods, I recommend oils because they contain a higher concentration of the needed nutrients.

RECOMMENDED HERBS	RECOMMENDED FOODS
Corn Silk	Beef
Echinacea Angustifolia	Cacao
Fennel	Canola Oil
Ginger	Cayenne Pepper
Plantain	Cinnamon
Uva Ursi	Eggs
Valerian Root	Milk
Witch Hazel	Olive Oil
Yerba Santa	Peanut Oil
Yucca	Raspberries
	Salmonberries
	Sesame Oil
	Soy Oil
	Strawberries
	Sunflower Oil
	Walnut Oil

Recommended Herbs

Corn Silk

Latin: *Zea Mays*

Vitamins
N/A

Minerals
Potassium Chloride

Trace Minerals
Vanadium

Amino Acids
Threonine
Tyrosine

Phenolics
Urushiol
Valeric Acid
Vanillylamine
Xanthine

Metabolic Enzymes
Urokinase

Digestive Enzymes
Intrinsic Factor

Echinacea Angustifolia

Latin: *Echinacea Angustifolia*

Vitamins
N/A

Minerals
Zinc Sulfate

Trace Minerals
Vanadium

Amino Acids
N/A

Phenolics
Vanillic Acid
Vanillylamine
Xanthine

Metabolic Enzymes
Urokinase

Digestive Enzymes
N/A

Fennel

Latin: *Foeniculum Vulgare*

Vitamins
Inositol

Minerals
Sodium Chloride

Trace Minerals
Silicon

Amino Acids
Tryptophan

Phenolics
Gallic Acid
Vanillic Acid
Vanillin
Vanillylamine
Xanthine

Metabolic Enzymes
Phosphomannose Isomerase

Digestive Enzymes
N/A

Ginger

Latin: *Zingiber Officinale*

Vitamins
Inositol

Minerals
Sodium Chloride

Trace Minerals
Silicon

Amino Acids
Tryptophan

Phenolics
Gallic Acid
Vanillic Acid
Vanillin
Vanillylamine
Xanthine

Metabolic Enzymes
Phosphomannose Isomerase

Digestive Enzymes
Amylase
Cellulase
Intrinsic Factor
Maltase

Plantain

Latin: *Plantago Major*

Vitamins
N/A

Minerals
Potassium Chloride

Trace Minerals
Vanadium

Amino Acids
Threonine
Tyrosine

Phenolics
Vanillylamine
Xanthine

Metabolic Enzymes
Baker's Yeast Enzyme
Urokinase

Digestive Enzymes
N/A

Uva Ursi

Latin: *Arctostaphylos Uva Ursi*

Vitamins
N/A

Minerals
N/A

Trace Minerals
Selenium

Amino Acids
Threonine

Phenolics
Vanillin
Vanillylamine
Xanthine

Metabolic Enzymes
SOD (Superoxide Dismutase)

Digestive Enzymes
N/A

Valerian Root

Latin: *Valeriana Officinalis*

Vitamins
N/A

Minerals
Sodium Chloride

Trace Minerals
N/A

Amino Acids
N/A

Phenolics
Valeric Acid
Vanillic Acid
Vanillin
Vanillylamine
Xanthine

Metabolic Enzymes
Baker's Yeast Enzyme

Digestive Enzymes
N/A

Witch Hazel

Latin: *Hamamelis Virginiana*

Vitamins
N/A

Minerals
Sodium Chloride

Trace Minerals
Titanium

Amino Acids
Tyrosine

Phenolics
Vanillic Acid
Vanillin
Vanillylamine
Xanthine

Metabolic Enzymes
Baker's Yeast Enzyme
Urokinase

Digestive Enzymes
Intrinsic Factor

Yerba Santa

Latin: *Eriodictyon Californicum*

Vitamins
N/A

Minerals
Zinc Sulfate

Trace Minerals
Vanadium

Amino Acids
N/A

Phenolics
Vanillic Acid
Vanillylamine
Xanthine

Metabolic Enzymes
Urokinase

Digestive Enzymes
Intrinsic Factor

Yucca

Latin: Yucca *Filimentosa*

Vitamins
N/A

Minerals
N/A

Trace Minerals
Selenium

Amino Acids
Threonine

Phenolics
Vanillin
Vanillylamine
Xanthine

Metabolic Enzymes
SOD (Superoxide Dismutase)

Digestive Enzymes
Intrinsic Factor

Recommended Foods

Before listing the nutrients in foods that I have found to be necessary for detoxification, I want to make a comment about the importance of digestive enzymes. Notice the nutrients found in the herbs Echinacea, Uva Ursi, and Fennel, then compare them to the nutrients found in Yerba Santa, Yucca, and Ginger. The cofactors are identical. The only difference is that Yerba Santa, Yucca, and Ginger all contain digestive enzymes. Echinacea, Uva Ursi, and Fennel do not contain any digestive enzymes.

What this means is that Yerba Santa, Yucca, and Ginger work much better at detoxification than the other three herbs. I have found through using these herbs that they do work faster and more efficiently simply because they contain digestive enzymes. The other three herbs do work, and may be easier to find in health food stores, but my point is that herbs work much better if they not only contain the necessary metabolic enzymes, but also digestive enzymes. Remember, enzymes are the delivery mechanism, and the right delivery increases the effectiveness of the herbs.

Beef

Vitamins
Vitamin B3 (Niacin)*
Vitamin C*
Inositol

Minerals
Iron*
Magnesium*
Potassium Chloride
Sodium Chloride

Trace Minerals
Vanadium

Amino Acids
Threonine
Tyrosine

Phenolics
Valeric Acid
Vanillic Acid
Xanthine

Metabolic Enzymes
N/A

Digestive Enzymes
Ribonuclease

*Component not directly involved with detoxification.

Cacao

Vitamins
N/A

Minerals
Magnesium*

Trace Minerals
Selenium
Titanium
Vanadium

Amino Acids
N/A

Phenolics
Vanillic Acid
Xanthine

Metabolic Enzymes
Baker's Yeast Enzyme

Digestive Enzymes
Bromelain
Cellulase
Lipase
Papain
Pepsin
Protease
Ribonuclease
Trypsin

*Component not directly involved with detoxification.

Canola Oil

Vitamins
N/A

Minerals
Calcium*
Sodium Chloride

Trace Minerals
Vanadium

Amino Acids
Tryptophan
Tyrosine

Phenolics
Vanillic Acid
Vanillin
Vanillylamine
Xanthine

Metabolic Enzymes
Urokinase

Digestive Enzymes
N/A

*Component not directly involved with detoxification.

Cayenne Pepper

Vitamins
N/A

Minerals
Potassium Chloride
Zinc Sulfate

Trace Minerals
Silicon
Vanadium

Amino Acids
N/A

Phenolics
Quercetin*
Vanillic Acid
Vanillylamine
Xanthine

Metabolic Enzymes
Urokinase

Digestive Enzymes
Maltase
Potassium Bicarbonate
Protease
Sodium Bicarbonate

*Component not directly involved with detoxification.

Cinnamon

Vitamins
N/A

Minerals
Potassium Chloride
Zinc Sulfate

Trace Minerals
Silicon
Titanium

Amino Acids
Threonine

Phenolics
Gallic Acid
Vanillic Acid
Vanillylamine
Xanthine

Metabolic Enzymes
Urokinase

Digestive Enzymes
Maltase
Pepsin
Potassium Bicarbonate

Eggs

Vitamins
N/A

Minerals
Calcium*
Potassium Chloride
Sodium Chloride
Zinc Sulfate

Trace Minerals
Selenium
Titanium

Amino Acids
Taurine*

Phenolics
Coumarin
Gallic Acid
Urushiol
Vanillin
Vanillylamine
Xanthine

Metabolic Enzymes
N/A

Digestive Enzymes
Cellulase
Maltase
Ribonuclease

*Component not directly involved with detoxification.

Milk

Vitamins
N/A

Minerals
Calcium Lactate*
Sodium Chloride

Trace Minerals
Silicon

Amino Acids
Tryptophan

Phenolics
Gallic Acid
Xanthine

Metabolic Enzymes
N/A

Digestive Enzymes
Lactase*
Ribonuclease

*Component not directly involved with detoxification.

Olive Oil

Vitamins
N/A

Minerals
Potassium*

Trace Minerals
Selenium

Amino Acids
N/A

Phenolics
Xanthine

Metabolic Enzymes
Baker's Yeast Enzyme

Digestive Enzymes
N/A

*Component not directly involved with detoxification.

Peanut Oil

Vitamins
Inositol

Minerals
Sodium Chloride

Trace Minerals
Silicon

Amino Acids
Tryptophan

Phenolics
Gallic Acid
Vanillic Acid
Vanillin
Vanillylamine
Xanthine

Metabolic Enzymes
Phosphomannose Isomerase

Digestive Enzymes
Amylase
Cellulase
Intrinsic Factor
Maltase

Raspberries (Red)

Vitamins
N/A

Minerals
N/A

Trace Minerals
N/A

Amino Acids
N/A

Phenolics
N/A

Metabolic Enzymes
Phosphomannose Isomerase
Urokinase

Digestive Enzymes
Amylase
Bromelain
Cellulase
Intrinsic Factor
Lipase
Maltase
Ribonuclease
Pancreatin
Potassium Bicarbonate
Protease
Trypsin

Salmonberries

Vitamins
Inositol

Minerals
N/A

Trace Minerals
N/A

Amino Acids
N/A

Phenolics
Xanthine

Metabolic Enzymes
N/A

Digestive Enzymes
Bromelain
Intrinsic Factor
Maltase

Sesame Oil

Vitamins
N/A

Minerals
Sodium Chloride

Trace Minerals
Titanium

Amino Acids
Tyrosine

Phenolics
Vanillic Acid
Vanillin
Vanillylamine
Xanthine

Metabolic Enzymes
Baker's Yeast Enzyme
Urokinase

Digestive Enzymes
Intrinsic Factor

Soy Oil

Vitamins
N/A

Minerals
Sodium Chloride

Trace Minerals
Titanium

Amino Acids
Tyrosine

Phenolics
Vanillylamine

Metabolic Enzymes
SOD (Superoxide Dismutase)

Digestive Enzymes
N/A

Strawberries

Vitamins
N/A

Minerals
N/A

Trace Minerals
N/A

Amino Acids
N/A

Phenolics
Valeric Acid
Xanthine

Metabolic Enzymes
Baker's Yeast Enzyme
Phosphomannose Isomerase
SOD (Superoxide Dismutase)

Digestive Enzymes
Amylase
Bromelain
Cellulase
Intrinsic Factor
Lipase
Maltase
Ribonuclease
Pancreatin
Papain
Pepsin
Protease
Sodium Bicarbonate
Trypsin

Sunflower Oil

Vitamins
N/A

Minerals
Iron*
Magnesium*
Potassium Chloride

Trace Minerals
Vanadium

Amino Acids
Threonine
Tyrosine

Phenolics
Urushiol
Valeric Acid
Vanillylamine
Xanthine

Metabolic Enzymes
Urokinase

Digestive Enzymes
Amylase
Intrinsic Factor
Lipase
Pancreatin
Protease
Trypsin

*Component not directly involved with detoxification.

Walnut Oil

Vitamins
N/A

Minerals
Potassium Chloride
Zinc Sulfate

Trace Minerals
Vanadium

Amino Acids
Threonine
Tyrosine

Phenolics
Vanillic Acid
Vanillin
Xanthine

Metabolic Enzymes
Baker's Yeast Enzyme

Digestive Enzymes
Amylase
Bromelain
Lipase
Pancreatin
Papain
Pepsin
Potassium Bicarbonate
Protease
Ribonuclease
Sodium Bicarbonate
Trypsin

NUTRIENT SUPERSTARS

As humans, we are limited by how many calories we can consume on a daily basis. As a result, I believe we should limit our calories to the foods which contain the highest levels of nutrients. I have chosen just a few herbs and foods in this next list that have the very highest levels of enzymes and cofactors.

Through my testing, I have found that there are five herbs which contain the very highest milligramsof metabolic enzymes and cofactors needed daily for detoxifying: Corn Silk, Ginger, Witch Hazel, Yerba Santa, and Yucca. I would say that typically, if one were to take 2–4 capsules daily, each containing 400–500 milligrams, that this would supply an adequate amount of metabolic enzymes and cofactors needed daily for detoxification.

The foods containing the very highest levels of cofactors are beef, milk, and eggs. The amount needed will vary according to each person's size, age, and physical activity. I would say that on average, the foods used as cofactors should make up about 50% of one's daily caloric intake. The remaining 50% should be made up of the foods containing the highest levels of metabolic and digestive enzymes.

The foods containing the highest levels of metabolic and digestive enzymes are strawberries, raspberries, and cacao. Strawberries and raspberries contain mostly carbohydrates, with very little protein and fat. Cacao seeds are mostly fat with some carbohydrates and protein. The daily intake of digestive enzymes needs to be an equal and balanced amount of each individual enzyme.

Assuming the average adult consumes 2,000 calories a day, then approximately two cups daily of strawberries and raspberries, with about three ounces of cacao would be a sufficient amount. This amount, divided between 2–3 meals daily, will vary according to size, age, and physical activity. A child would need ¼ to ½ the amount an adult would consume.

Nutrients To Eliminate Toxins

The following pages will list various toxin categories and what nutrients can be used to eliminate them.

TOXIN CATEGORIES

Parasites

Protozoa

Bacteria

Fungi

Viruses

Venoms

Chemicals

Medications

Vaccines

Heavy Metals

Radiation

The following are recommended in the treatment of Parasites:

Vitamins
N/A

Minerals
Potassium Chloride

Trace Minerals
Selenium
Vanadium

Amino Acids
Tyrosine

Phenolics
Vanillic Acid
Vanillylamine
Xanthine

Metabolic Enzymes
SOD (Superoxide Dismutase)

Digestive Enzymes
Intrinsic Factor

The following are recommended in the treatment of Protozoa:

Vitamins
N/A

Minerals
Potassium Chloride

Trace Minerals
Vanadium

Amino Acids
Threonine

Phenolics
Vanillic Acid
Xanthine

Metabolic Enzymes
Baker's Yeast Enzyme

Digestive Enzymes
Intrinsic Factor

The following are recommended in the treatment of Bacteria:

Vitamins
N/A

Minerals
Potassium Chloride

Trace Minerals
Vanadium

Amino Acids
N/A

Phenolics
Vanillic Acid
Xanthine

Metabolic Enzymes
SOD (Superoxide Dismutase)

Digestive Enzymes
Intrinsic Factor

The following are recommended in the treatment of Fungi:

Vitamins
N/A

Minerals
Sodium Chloride

Trace Minerals
Titanium

Amino Acids
N/A

Phenolics
Vanillic Acid
Xanthine

Metabolic Enzymes
Baker's Yeast Enzyme

Digestive Enzymes
Intrinsic Factor

The following are recommended in the treatment of Viruses:

Vitamins
N/A

Minerals
Zinc Sulfate

Trace Minerals
Vanadium

Amino Acids
Threonine

Phenolics
Valeric Acid
Vanillic Acid
Vanillylamine
Xanthine

Metabolic Enzymes
Urokinase

Digestive Enzymes
Intrinsic Factor

The following are recommended in the treatment of Venoms:

Vitamins
N/A

Minerals
Potassium Chloride

Trace Minerals
Vanadium

Amino Acids
N/A

Phenolics
Vanillylamine
Xanthine

Metabolic Enzymes
Baker's Yeast Enzyme

Digestive Enzymes
Intrinsic Factor

The following are recommended in the treatment of Chemicals:

Vitamins
N/A

Minerals
Potassium Chloride

Trace Minerals
Silicon

Amino Acids
Threonine

Phenolics
Vanillylamine
Xanthine

Metabolic Enzymes
Baker's Yeast Enzyme

Digestive Enzymes
Intrinsic Factor
Maltase

The following are recommended in the treatment of Medication Residue:

Vitamins
N/A

Minerals
Potassium Chloride

Trace Minerals
Selenium

Amino Acids
Threonine

Phenolics
Vanillylamine
Xanthine

Metabolic Enzymes
Baker's Yeast Enzyme

Digestive Enzymes
Intrinsic Factor
Maltase

The following are recommended in the treatment of Vaccine Residue:

Vitamins
Inositol

Minerals
Sodium Chloride

Trace Minerals
Vanadium

Amino Acids
N/A

Phenolics
Gallic Acid
Urushiol
Valeric Acid
Vanillic Acid
Vanillylamine
Xanthine

Metabolic Enzymes
Urokinase

Digestive Enzymes
Intrinsic Factor
Maltase
Trypsin

The following are recommended in the treatment of Heavy Metals:

Vitamins
Inositol

Minerals
Potassium Chloride
Zinc Sulfate

Trace Minerals
Silicon

Amino Acids
Tryptophan

Phenolics
Xanthine

Metabolic Enzymes
SOD (Superoxide Dismutase)

Digestive Enzymes
Intrinsic Factor

The following are recommended in the treatment of Radiation Residue:

Vitamins
N/A

Minerals
Potassium Chloride

Trace Minerals
Titanium

Amino Acids
Tyrosine

Phenolics
Vanillin
Xanthine

Metabolic Enzymes
Phosphomannose Isomerase

Digestive Enzymes
Intrinsic Factor

FINAL THOUGHTS

Being physically ill can, and usually does, have a devastating affect on a person's mental state. I have always found it more difficult to deal with my illnesses mentally than physically. Many times I have felt like I was at the mercy of the elements. For example, if I was in a house, building, or just a room that smelled of mold, mildew, or being musty, I felt a fear come over me because I knew I would probably start having trouble breathing soon due to my history with asthma. I would also fear pollen season, especially in the evenings when the air is heavier with humidity.

During the winter months, when the weather turned colder and the air dryer, I always felt like I was such a victim to my environment. This would be the time of year when my skin would become much dryer and itch. I would also get cracks on my fingers and the bottoms of my feet that would sometimes bleed and be extremely painful. Working with my hands, or just walking around were difficult and painful. My symptoms increased so slowly over time that I finally considered this pattern of decreasing health normal for me. I could no longer do many things that I had once been able to enjoy. I felt alone and isolated from others who were healthier, or at least who I viewed to be healthier. I was afraid that if they knew my health situation they would certainly reject me. I desperately wanted to live a normal life and not have to worry about my health. Other people seemed to be able to do and eat whatever they wanted to with no consequences. I was envious of their freedom.

My feelings of isolation and fear of possible ridicule left me in a mental state that invariably increased my physical symptoms. We all want to be healthy and happy. Humans are social creatures and need contact with others. When we feel separation from others, this causes a negative state of mind which can make us feel worse physically. Our brains are trainable. Our bodies will manifest what our mind focuses on. If we focus on all the negatives in our life, we will continue to see more and more negative, and risk manifesting illness and disease in our bodies. If we focus on the good in our life, we will continue to see more and more of the positive, manifesting health and harmony in our bodies.

I can certainly understand why people choose to take traditional medications to relieve their symptoms. It seems so easy to take a pill to mask symptoms in order to enjoy life. The only problem with this is that over time the symptoms usually get worse, requiring more pills, or stronger pills, or even several medications. With this book, I hope to offer another option: eliminate the root cause of the symptoms, so the symptoms can be eliminated permanently.

With my research and resulting change in diet, I no longer need to fear musty-smelling rooms or pollen season because my symptoms are eliminated. This is what I want for everyone else, too. It does no good for our society, or the world in general, for people to suffer. I want people to live happy, healthy lives and accomplish great things with their God-given gifts and talents. I want people to have healthy bodies and positive states of mind. Time should be spent appreciating the beauty in life, rather than wasting time with worry and fear.

In fifteen years of practice, I have tested thousands of people. I say practice, because the study of the body is not an exact science. I have discovered a multitude of similarities, finding many of the same toxins in most people. I propose an open mind when considering my theories, just as open minds where needed when Aristotle first theorized the world was round, or when Iganz Semmelweis suggested that physicians should wash their hands between patients to lower mortality rates.

The Story of Ignaz Semmelweis

Ignaz Philipp Semmelweis was a Hungarian physician in the mid 1800's. Puerperal fever, also called childbed fever, was common at that time. It was often fatal, with a mortality rate of 10% - 35%, often affecting women shortly after childbirth.

Many women knew this and thus preferred to give birth on the street rather than risking the obstetric clinics. The medical establishment believed that Puerperal fever was non-preventable. The scientific opinion of that time was the belief that diseases were caused by an imbalance in human temperament, a theory known as dyscrasia.

During this period, it was a common medical practice for doctors to move directly from one patient to the next without washing their hands. They would even perform autopsies on diseased bodies and then move directly on to examining living patients without any hygienic preparation.

Semmelweis, as head of the Vienna General Hospital's First Obstetric Clinic, postulated the theory that particles introduced into the women caused Puerperal fever. The breakthrough for his theory occurred in 1847 when his physician friend, Jacob Kolletschka, died from an infection contracted after his finger was accidentally punctured with a knife during a routine autopsy. Kolletschka's own autopsy revealed a disease condition similar to that of women who contracted Puerperal fever.

Semmelweis hypothesized that there was a connection between contamination from cadavers in autopsies and Puerperal fever. He made a detailed study of mortality statistics in his own clinic and concluded that doctors and medical students carried infecting particles on their hands from the autopsy room to their patients in the obstetric clinic.

At that time, there was no knowledge of antiseptics and patients were subject to overcrowding and the use of contaminated instruments, dressings and bedding. The germ theory of disease was not developed until 1879 by Louis Pasteur. Semmelweis concluded that some unknown "cadaver substance" caused Puerperal fever and ordered that hands and instruments be washed with a chlorinated lime solution before all examinations.

Even though mortality rates quickly dropped from over 18% to just over 1%, his findings were rejected by much of the medical establishment. Doctors argued that even if his findings were correct, washing one's hands each time before treating patients would be too much work.

Some were even quoted as saying such things as, "Doctors are gentlemen, and gentlemen's hands are clean." Also, the medical establishment was reluctant to accept that they had themselves caused so many deaths.

Semmelweis' claims were also rejected because no scientific explanation could be given as proof. One of Semmelweis' supporters wrote two articles on his behalf, and although many foreign physicians were impressed by his apparent discovery, in 1849 he was still fired from his position in Vienna. It would be decades before Louis Pasteur could offer proof of his findings.

He returned to Hungary to take charge of the maternity ward of a hospital where his hygiene protocols reduced the local mortality rate from Puerperal fever to less than 1%. In 1861 he published a book describing his findings and recommendations. He sent copies to medical societies in Germany, France, and England.

A number of unfavorable reviews came out on his book and most physicians rejected his ideas. The medical establishment's failure to recognize his findings led to the tragic and unnecessary death of thousands of patients.[80]

CONCLUSION

Throughout history, humans have been plagued by many diseases such as Leprosy, the Bubonic Plague, Smallpox, and Cholera.

Each of these diseases has one thing in common, a toxin as a root cause. Somewhere along the way we stopped eliminating toxins and started medicating symptoms because there is more money in treating the symptoms. Something is definitely wrong with this picture. My belief is that most diseases are caused by toxins, or in many cases, a combination of several toxins. I have repeatedly found that if toxins are removed from the body, symptoms disappear because the root cause has been eliminated.

Many bacterial diseases are no longer feared because antibiotics have been proven to cure them. The same can happen for a multitude of other diseases if we work on finding cures instead of just treatments. The root cause or toxin needs to be discovered and dealt with by a change in diet and supplementation of enzymes and co-factors.

In conclusion, I would like to say that much of what I have stated in this book is my opinion and supported solely by my own research. I am confident in my research because of the results I have witnessed in myself and in a multitude of patients over the years.

Using the right herbs, in the correct combinations, and at the proper milligrams, has shown to produce amazing results. For years I used homeopathics to detoxify myself. This was a long, frustrating period. The homeopathic approach is effective, and does work, but it is slow and inefficient. Herbs, on the other hand, are both effective and efficient.

My goal for writing this book has been to inform and guide the reader toward a better understanding of the role toxins play in our symptoms and diseases, as well as how to overcome them. My goal is to eliminate unnecessary human suffering by using herbal detoxification, the safest and most effective treatment I know.

REFERENCES

1. Dr. Voll. Page: 14
   http://www.biomeridian.com/voll.html
   http://www.diamondhead.net/eav.html
   http://www.eavnet.com
   http://www.holistic-physician.com

2. Parasites-Nematodes, Cestodes, Trematodes. Page: 24
   The Merck Manual. Merck & Co., Inc., 2005.
   Gittleman, Ann Loise, *Guess What Came to Dinner: Parasites and your health*, Avery, 1993.
   Kroeger, Hanna, Parasites: The Enemy Within, 1991.

3. Neurotransmitters and Amino Acids. Page: 27
   http://www.vitamins-supplements.org

4. Leptospirosis, Lyme, Syphilis. Pages: 27
   Saunders Comprehensive Veterinary Dictionary, Third Edition, D.C. Blood, V.P. Studdert and C.C. Gay, Elsevier, 2007.

5. Autism. Page: 29
   The Merck Manual. Merck & Co., Inc., 1999.
   Gale Encyclopedia of Neurological Disorders. The Gale Group, Inc., 2005
   Children's Health Encyclopedia. Through a partnership of Answers Corporation., 2006.

6. Venoms-Hemotoxic & Nerotoxic. Page: 31
   The American Heritage Stedman's Medical Dictionary, Houghton Mifflin Company, 2002.

7. Pesticides. Page: 33
   http://www.epa.gov
   http://www.purdue.edu

8. Recombinant DNA. Page: 33
   Garret, R.H. & Grisham, C.M., *Biochemistry.*, Saunders College Publishers, 2000.
   Colowick, S.P. & Kapian, O.N., *Methods in Enzymology*, Volume 68; Recombinant DNA, Academic Press, 1980.

9. Free Radical Reactions with Heavy Metals. Page: 34
   The Columbia Electronic Encyclopedia, Sixth Edition, Columbia University Press, 2003.

10. Homeopathy-Nosodes, Isodes, Sarcodes. Page: 41
    D.C. Blood, V.P. Studdert and C.C. Gay, *Saunders Comprehensive Veterinary Dictionary*, Third Edition, Elsevier, 2007.
    http://www.tcfnm.com/homeopathy.htm

11. Amplitude and Energy. Page: 42
    The Science of Everyday Things. The Gale Group, Inc., 2002.

12. Resonance. Page: 42
    Gerber, Richard, *Vibrational Medicine: New Choices for Healing Ourselves,* Bear & Co.; Updated Edition, 1996.

13. Definition of Herxheimer Reaction. Page: 43
    http://www.falconblanco.com/health/crisis.html
    The American Heritage Stedman's Medical Dictionary, Houghton Mifflin Company, 2002.
    http://www.silver-colloids.com/Pubs/herxheimer.html

14 Endotoxins. Page: 43
    McGraw-Hill Encyclopedia of Science and Technology,
    The Mcgraw-Hill Companies, Inc., 2005.

15 Quinine/Malaria. Page: 44
    Britannica Concise Encyclopedia. Encyclopedia Britannica,
    Inc., 2006.
    McGraw-Hill Encyclopedia of Science And Technology,
    The Mcgraw-Hill Companies, Inc., 2005.

16 Definition of Metabolic Enzymes. Page : 46
    http://www.answers.com/topic/metabolic-enzyme

17 Cofactors and Coenzymes. Page : 46
    Britannica Concise Encyclopedia. Encyclopedia Britannica,
    Inc., 2006.

18 Metabolic Enzymes. Page : 47
    http://www.enzymedica.com
    http://www.hepatitis-c.de/enzyme.htm

19 Carbohydrate-deficient Glycoprotein Syndrome Type Ib.
    Page : 47
    http://www.jci.org

20 Phytochemicals. Page : 49
    McGraw-Hill Encyclopedia of Science and Technology,
    The Mcgraw-Hill Companies, Inc., 2005.
    Food and Fitness: A Dictionary of Diet And Exercise.,
    Oxford University Press, 2003.

21 Homeopathy/Miasms. Page : 51
    Hahnemann, Samuel, *Chronic Diseases*, 1828.
    The Oxford Companion to the Body., Oxford University
    Press., 2003.
    Encyclopedia of Alternative Medicine., The Gale Group,
    Inc., 2005.

22 Teratology. Page : 51
   Human Embryology & Teratology., New York Wiley-Liss, 2001.

23 Thalidomide. Page : 51
   http://www.thalidomide.ca/en/index.html

24 Diethylstilbesterol. Page : 52
   http://www.autoimmunedisease.suite101.com

25 Foetal Damage & Birth Defects. Page : 52
   http://www.whale.to/vaccines/foetal.html
   http://www.pediatrics.about.com

26 Thyroid, Pituitary, Hypothalamus. Page : 53
   The Oxford Companion to the Body., Oxford University Press., 2003.

27 Intrinsic Factor Deficiency; IDF. Page : 65
   http://www.ncbi.nlm.nih.gov
   The Intrinsic Factor is Vital for B12 Absorption.
      http://www.findarticles.com
   Congenital Lack of Intrinsic Factor.
      http://www.healthdiscovery.com

28 Essential amino acids. Page : 70
   The Oxford Dictionary of Sports Science and Medicine., Michael Kent, 2007.

29 Intelligence of the human brain, and diet. Page : 71
   http://www.beyondveg.com

30 Skin and the aging process. Page : 74
   http://www.mirabellaskincare.com
   http://www.geocites.com

31 Enzymes. Page : 88
   http://www.geocities.com

32 Apoenzymes and Holoenzymes. Page : 89
    The American Heritage Stedman's Medical Dictionary, Houghton Mifflin Company, 2002.

33 Digestive Enzymes. Page : 90
    http://www.enzymedica.com

34 Amylase. Page : 91
    http://www.britannica.com
    McGraw-Hill Encyclopedia of Science and Technology, The Mcgraw-Hill Companies, Inc., 2005.

35 Bromelain. Page : 92
    A Dictionary of Food and Nutrition. A.E. Bender and D.A. Bender, 2005.
    Encyclopedia of Alternative Medicine., The Gale Group, Inc., 2005.

36 Cellulase. Page : 93
    http://www.worthington-biochem.com

37 Intrinsic Factor Page : 94
    Food and Fitness: A Dictionary of Diet And Exercise., Oxford University Press, 2003.
    http://www.vivo.colostate.edu

38 Lipase. Page : 95
    The Oxford Dictionary of Sports Science, Oxford University Press, 2007.

39 Maltase. Page : 96
    The American Heritage Dictionary of the English Language, Fourth Edition, Houghton Mifflin Company, 2007.

40 Pancreatin. Page : 97
    The American Heritage Dictionary of the English Language, Fourth Edition, Houghton Mifflin Company, 2007.

41 Papain. Page : 98
The American Heritage Dictionary of the English Language, Fourth Edition, Houghton Mifflin Company, 2007.
A Dictionary of Food and Nutrition. A.E. Bender and D.A. Bender, 2005.
Encyclopedia of Alternative Medicine., The Gale Group, Inc., 2005.

42 Pepsin. Page : 99
McGraw-Hill Encyclopedia of Science and Technology, The Mcgraw-Hill Companies, Inc., 2005.
Britannica Concise Encyclopedia, Encyclopedia Britannica, Inc., 2006.

43 Potassium Bicarbonate. Page : 100
http//www.epa.gov

44 Protease. Page : 101
Barrett, A.J., Rawlings ND, Woessner JF. *The Handbook of Proteolytic Enzymes.*, Second Edition, Academic Press, 2003.

45 Ribonuclease. Page : 102
http://www.iscid.org
McGraw-Hill Encyclopedia of Science and Technology, The Mcgraw-Hill Companies, Inc., 2005.

46 Sodium Bicarbonate. Page : 103
McGraw-Hill Encyclopedia of Science and Technology, The Mcgraw-Hill Companies, Inc., 2003.
The Columbia Electronic Encyclopedia, Sixth Edition, Columbia University Press, 2003.

47 Trypsin. Page : 104
The Columbia Electronic Encyclopedia, Sixth Edition, Columbia University Press, 2003.

48 Enzymes. Page : 105
    The Oxford Companion to the Body. Oxford University Press., 2003.

49 Mannose phosphate isomerase. Page : 106
    http://www.nlm.nih.gov

50 CDGS. Page : 106
    http://www.aacpdm.org
    http://www.tmri.org

51 SOD. Page : 107
    http://www.3dchem.com
    http://www.worthington-biochem.com
    http://www.nature.com

52 Urokinase. Page : 108
    http://www.drugs.com.
    http://www.ncbi.nhl.nih.gov
    http://www.sciencemag.org

53 Baker's yeast. Page : 109
    http://www.phys.ksu.edu/gene/a1.html

54 Baker's Yeast Enzyme. Page : 109
    http://www.ncbi.nlm.gov
    http://www3.interscience.wiley.com
    http://wwwjbc.org

55 Vitamins. Page : 111
    The American Heritage Dictionary of the English Language, Fourth Edition, Houghton Mifflin Company, 2007.
    McGraw-Hill Encyclopedia of Science and Technology, The Mcgraw-Hill Companies, Inc., 2005.

56 Coenzymes. Page : 112
    McGraw-Hill Encyclopedia of Science and Technology, The Mcgraw-Hill Companies, Inc., 2005.

57 Inositol. Page : 113
Merck Index. Merck & Co., Inc., Eleventh Edition, 1989.

58 Minerals. Page : 116
The Columbia Electronic Encyclopedia, Sixth Edition, Columbia University Press, 2003.
http://www.portfolio.mvm.ed.ac.uk

59 Potassium Chloride. Page : 117
Handbook of Chemistry and Physics. 71st Edition, CRC Press, 1990.

60 Sodium Chloride. Page : 118
Encyclopedia of Chemical Technology. John Wiley and Sons, Inc., 2005.
Britannica Concise Encyclopedia, Encyclopedia Britannica, Inc., 2006.

61 Zinc Sulfate. Page : 119
The Columbia Electronic Encyclopedia, Sixth Edition, Columbia University Press, 2003.

62 Trace Elements. Page : 121
http://www.healthgoods.com
The Concise Oxford Dictionary of Archeology. Oxford University Press, 2003.
Encyclopedia of Food and Culture, The Gale Group, Inc., 2003.

63 Selenium. Page : 123
A Dictionary of Food and Nutrition. A.E. Bender and D.A. Bender, 2003.

64 Silicon. Page : 124
The Columbia Electronic Encyclopedia, Sixth Edition, Columbia University Press, 2003.

65 Titanium. Page : 125
Britannica Concise Encyclopedia. Encyclopedia Britannica, Inc., 2006.

66 Vanadium. Page : 126
McGraw-Hill Encyclopedia of Science and Technology, The Mcgraw-Hill Companies, Inc., 2005.
Encyclopedia of Alternative Medicine. The Gale Group, Inc., 2005.

67 Amino Acids. Page : 128
Science of Everyday Things. The Gale Group, Inc., 2002.
McGraw-Hill Encyclopedia of Science and Technology, The Mcgraw-Hill Companies, Inc., 2005.
http://www.cocoonnutrition.org

68 Threonine. Page : 129
Principles of Biochemistry. Lehninger, Third Edition, Worth Publishing, New York, 2000.

69 Tryptophan. Page : 130
A Dictionary of Food and Nutrition. A.E. Bender and D.A. Bender, 2003.
Food and Fitness: A Dictionary of Diet and Exercise, Oxford Univerity Press, 2003.
The American Heritage Dictionary of the English Language, Fourth Edition, Houghton Mifflin Company, 2007.

70 Tyrosine. Page : 131
The American Heritage Dictionary of the English Language, Fourth Edition, Houghton Mifflin Company, 2007.
Mosby's Dental Dictionary, Elsevier, Inc., 2004.

71 Phytonutrients. Page : 134
   http://www.ars.usda.gov
   Food and Fitness: A Dictionary of Diet and Exercise, Oxford University Press, 2003.
   The Oxford Dictionary of Sports Science & Medicine., Michael Kent, 2007.
   http://www.nutrifruit.com

72 Gallic Acid. Page : 135
   http://www.phytochemicals.info
   LD Reynolds and NG Wilson, "*Scribes and Scholars*" Third Edition, Oxford, 1991.

73 Urushiol. Page : 136
   The American Heritage Dictionary Of the English Language, Fourth Edition, Houghton Mifflin Company, 2007.
   The American Heritage Stedman's Medical Dictionary, Houghton Mifflin Company, 2002.

74 Valeric Acid. Page : 137
   The Merck Index. Merck & Co., Inc., Twelfth Edition, 1996.

75 Vanillic Acid. Page : 138
   http://www.chemicalland21.com

76 Vanillin. Page : 139
   Kirk-Othmer, *Encyclopedia of Chemical Technology.*, Third Edition, New York: John Wiley & Sons, 1983.

77 Vanillylamine. Page : 140
   The American Heritage Dictionary Of the English Language, Fourth Edition, Houghton Mifflin Company, 2007.

78 Alkaloid. Page : 141
    http://www.ansci.cornell.edu
    Organic Chemistry, Sixth Edition, New York, McGraw Hill, 2006.

79 Xanthine. Page : 141
    Merck Index. Merck & Co., Inc., Eleventh Edition, 1989.
    Saunders Comprehensive Veterinary Dictionary, Third Edition, Elsevier, 2007.

80 Ignaz Philipp Semmelweis. Page : 191
    http://www.Concise.Britannica.com
    Betrayers of the Truth:Fraud and Deceit In the Halls of Science., Simon and Schuster, NY; 1982.